Clinical Skills in Nursing

Also by Maggie Nicol (with Jane Dacre):

Clinical Skills: The Learning Matrix for Students of Medicine and Nursing (Radcliffe Medical Press, 1996)

Clinical Skills in Nursing

The return of the practical room?

Edited by

Maggie Nicol

and

Sally Glen

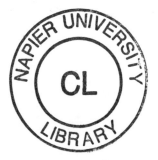

MACMILLAN

CA

First published 1999 by
MACMILLAN PRESS LTD
Houndmills, Basingstoke, Hampshire RG21 6XS
and London
Companies and representatives throughout the world

ISBN 0–333–72614–6 paperback

A catalogue record for this book is available from the British Library.

This book is printed on paper suitable for recycling and made from fully managed and sustained forest sources.

10 9 8 7 6 5 4 3 2 1
08 07 06 05 04 03 02 01 00 99

Editing and origination by
Aardvark Editorial, Mendham, Suffolk

Printed in Hong Kong

Contents

List of Contributors

Rosemary Allen MSc, BSc(Hons), DipN (Part A), RNT, RCNT, RGN is a Senior Lecturer within the Faculty of Health, University of Central Lancashire.

Carol Bavin RGN, RM, RCNT, DN is a Lecturer at St Bartholomew School of Nursing and Midwifery, City University, London.

Sally Glen MA(Ed), MA(Philosophy), DipEd(Lond), DipNEd, DN(Lond), RN, RSCN, RNT is Professor of Nursing Education, Dean of School of Nursing and Midwifery, University of Dundee.

Beryl Howard RN, MSc(Nurs), DipN(Lond), RCNT, RNT is Director of Pre-Registration Education at the Department of Nursing, Faculty of Healthcare and Social Work Studies, University of Salford.

Dorothy Jones MA, BEd(Hons), RNT, RN is Principal Lecturer at the Department of Primary and Community Nursing, University of Central Lancashire.

Iain McA Ledingham MBChB, MD(Hons), FRCS(Edin), FRCP(Edin/Glas), FInstBiol, FCCM, FRSE is Professor of Medical Education, Director of Clinical Skills Centre, Medical School, University of Dundee.

Maggie Nicol BSc(Hons), MSc, RGN, DN, PGDip(Ed) is a Senior Lecturer in Clinical Skills at St Bartholomew School of Nursing and Midwifery, City University, London.

Karen Veitch MSc, BSc, RGN, DN is a Practice Development Co-ordinator at the Primary Care Development Centre, Newcastle Upon Tyne.

Isabelle Whaite MA, DPSN, CertEd, RN, RM, RNT is a Principal Lecturer at the Faculty of Health, University of Central Lancashire.

Foreword

The past decade has seen a growing interest in the teaching and learning of clinical nursing skills by students, practitioners, nurse teachers, managers and policy makers.

Despite methodological differences, it is striking that similar themes and issues are emerging from the numerous evaluation studies carried out since the introduction of the Project 2000 pre-registration programmes in the UK. These are notably in the area of clinical skills acquisition and show that newly qualified nurses often lack competence in what are frequently basic, fundamental nursing skills. Clinical skills acquisition is, of course, an essential prerequisite for registration as a nurse and this state of what Luker *et al.* (1966)[1] refer to as 'practical skills illiteracy' is untenable.

In order to prepare future practitioners who are able to function effectively in a variety of healthcare settings, students now gain experience in a wide range of hospital and community placements. However, this means that they spend less time in a hospital ward setting, where students have traditionally developed and practised their skills. As nurse educators and healthcare providers struggle to identify sufficient quality clinical placements for increasingly large numbers of students, it is vital that students do not waste valuable clinical time learning how to perform fundamental nursing skills. That time should be spent practising and perfecting those skills, caring for real patients and clients with very real needs.

As the authors of this book argue, it is no longer sufficient to rely on students acquiring clinical skills by unstructured exposure in the placement. Skills teaching must be planned into the curriculum in order to prepare students for their placements so that they can optimise their learning within the context of an increasingly scarce and finite resource.

It is perhaps time, as the title of this book suggests, to reflect on the wisdom of removing the practical room from the educational base. Although at the time it appeared educationally sound to redirect the teaching of clinical skills to the patient at the bedside, it would seem that insufficient planning was undertaken to ensure that essential skills would be taught. With hind-sight, it is interesting to note that nursing chose to eschew the virtues of simulation at a time when other practice disciplines, notably airline pilots, were looking to the virtual reality of simu-lators to hone their skills. The concurrent demise of the clin-ical teacher role and the increase in the academic workload of the nurse teacher has left practitioners with a heavy responsi-bility for skills acquisition and assessment of competence.

This book examines the use of simulation in skills teaching and the introduction of a new kind of practical room, the clin-ical skills laboratory. With memories of run-down practical rooms full of out-of-date equipment still fresh in many people's minds, this may be viewed as a retrograde step. However, as this book illustrates, modern clinical skills laboratories are not simply a re-introduction of the practical room. They seek to provide a realistic simulation of clinical practice with up-to-date clinical equipment, opportunities for self-directed access by students, video recording and playback facilities, an approp-riate environment for realistic campus-based practical exami-nations, and opportunities for shared learning with other healthcare students. Used creatively by clinically competent academic staff in the ways described in this book, skills labor-atories will undoubtedly play an important part in the devel-opment of healthcare professionals of the future.

I am also pleased with the emphasis on shared learning with other clinicians. Healthcare is very much about teamwork, co-operation and collaboration. This needs to begin in the class-room or, rather, the skills laboratory. But clearly the skills laboratory is not a resource that should be restricted to the use of pre-registration students. The skills laboratory also has much to offer to continuing professional education and specialist training.

I commend this book to all involved in the education and training of healthcare professionals, be they academics, clini-cians or managers. It is indeed timely and much needed.

ANNE JARVIE
Chief Nursing Officer

[1] Luker, K., Carlisle, C., Riley, E., Stitwell, J., Davies C. and Wilson. R. (1966) *Project 2000 Fitness for Purpose, Report to the Department of Health*, University of Liverpool and University of Warwick.

Preface

The move to Diploma-level education that was achieved with
the introduction of Project 2000 has resulted in less time being
spent in clinical placements learning the art and science of
nursing. Clinical experience now extends into homes, factories, schools, shops and community agencies. Although the
integration of Colleges of Nursing and Midwifery into universities has undoubtedly invigorated the academic emphasis, it
has also led to concerns that newly qualified nurses are no longer
being equipped with the clinical skills that they need to fulfil
their professional role. The aim of this book is to bring together
current experience and future developments in clinical skills
teaching and learning, in particular the use of simulation and
nursing skills laboratories. It is intended to offer ideas and
practical guidance to those developing curricula in the changing
climate of health and social care provision.

Chapter 1 contextualises the debate related to clinical skills
acquisition by exploring the shift away from the traditional
apprentice-type model to a more education-led model of nurse
education. One response to the reduced exposure to real
patients and clients is to re-introduce the notion of the practical room and the use of simulated clinical practice to enable
students to develop fundamental nursing skills. Chapter 2
examines the strengths and limitations of the use of simulation and its potential application to nurse education. Chapter
3 describes how one school strengthened skills learning in the
curriculum, and outlines the development of a Clinical Skills
Centre. The discussion focuses on practical issues such as the
identification of resources; teaching, learning and assessment
strategies; and staff development issues.

In Chapter 4, the authors highlight the opportunities for
shared learning between nursing and medical students that
are made possible by the development of an interprofessional
skills teaching facility. The way in which student self-directed
learning in the Skills Centre is supported by 'in-house' instruc-

tional videos and workbooks, and the assessment of clinical skills using the Objective Structured Clinical Examination are also discussed.

Chapter 5 describes the ongoing development, implementation and evaluation of a multiprofessional Healthcare Learning Network. The concept is based on the premise that the development of knowledge, skills and attitudes is no longer bound in time and place but can occur at any time from any place. The Healthcare Learning Network is designed as a centre for learning with access and connectivity to resources well beyond the traditional physical constraints of a single building. The recruitment and training of members of the public to act as simulated patients to enable nursing, medical and other healthcare students to develop practical skills and problem identification and problem-solving abilities is also discussed.

Chapter 6 emphasises the importance of facilitating the integration of theory and practice through assessment strategies. The authors describe the use of a Portfolio as a tool for guiding and supporting learning in practice in order to develop professional competence. They describe how the Portfolio has provided a structured approach to skills teaching and learning that takes account of the reality of clinical practice. Chapter 7 expands the debate to include primary care personnel by describing an innovative resource centre designed to support and facilitate professional working in primary care. The author describes how the Skills Laboratory, which is part of the centre, helps primary care practitioners to address the difficulties experienced in clinical practice, such as acquiring specific technical skills, the organisation of training facilities and the provision of equipment. In the final chapter, the editors explore some issues currently influencing nurse education, for example the need to balance academic and clinical needs; the demand for multiprofessional education and practice; and the need to re-conceptualise the role of the nurse lecturer.

MAGGIE NICOL *City University*
SALLY GLEN *University of Dundee*

1

The Demise of the Apprenticeship Model

Sally Glen

Introduction

Until 1989, Registered General Nurse programmes were based on apprentice-type models, with much reliance upon experience gained in the clinical setting (traditionally the hospital) as a means of acquiring knowledge and skills. The first Diploma of Nursing in Higher Education (DipHE) (UKCC, 1986) courses in England commenced in September 1989, and the move of educational courses to Colleges of Nursing and Midwifery heralded the demise of traditional training courses centred in hospital Schools of Nursing. The merger and transfer of these Colleges into Universities in England, Scotland, Wales and Northern Ireland was completed in 1997.

Apprentice-type approaches

The combination of theoretical periods with associated practical experience, characterised by the pre-1989 training models, has much to commend it. This approach is supported by Gomez and Gomez (1987), who demonstrated that students learn quickly, and become more confident, from observing role models practising skills in clinical areas rather than in a classroom. Many nurse lecturers will verify this, but the research assumed structured supervision of experiences with time for reflection and not merely exposure to a clinical area (Studdy *et al.*, 1994). Apprentice-type models also rely heavily on the assumption that all clinical areas are staffed by highly competent and motivated staff who feel confident enough and have enough time to pass on their skills to student nurses. The adequacy of this model, with its assumption that qualified nurses would teach and supervise student nurses, has been questioned (Orton, 1981; Gott, 1983; Reid, 1985). The reality of service provision often thwarted the realisation of the advantages of an apprenticeship system. It has also been asserted that the emphasis upon the performance of activities, with little time for reflection, undermined the potential for learning (Chapman, 1980; UKCC, 1986; Greenwood, 1993).

Self-directed approaches

The volume and complexity of nursing knowledge has also continued to grow at an exponential rate. As Studdy *et al.* (1994) noted, the traditional pattern of nurse education, which relied heavily on teaching factual information and did not foster independent learning, critical reasoning or problem-solving among students, was inadequate and outmoded. Profound changes in the way in which we educate nurses were needed. A number of factors have contributed to the development of more flexible, self-directed approaches to learning in both nursing and higher education generally; these include globalisation, new technologies, an increasing demand on lecturers, the down-sizing of organisations, resource constraints and the concept of value for money. Flexible self-directed approaches are preferable to more traditional methods of teaching and learning that are more teacher centred in approach. There is also an assumption that nursing education should provide students with a variety of learning experiences and hence transferable skills. Transferable skills include problem-solving, verbal communication, self-enquiry, self-confidence, self-discipline and teamworking. The demand for transferable skills can be linked to changes that have taken place in industrial practice. The inability to work easily with other people as a member of a team is consistently identified by employers as being a deficit among British graduates (Levin, 1998).

Students needed therefore to become more responsible for their own learning and the acquisition of appropriate skills to support this. The purpose of getting students to participate in these kinds of activity is to encourage self-reliance and self-regulation. As nursing education has moved into the higher education sector, the demand to produce nurses with a high level of critical thinking and problem-solving skills (indicative of competent healthcare professionals) has increased. In addition, if we are to encourage creative, critical thinkers who can respond to the rapidly changing healthcare environment and the requirements of healthcare users, there is a need to promote independent activities in learners. Not surprisingly, self-directed learning is cited as a model of good educational practice (Knowles, 1990).

The advent of the diploma

The introduction of DipHE programmes offered students professional registration but also located nursing education completely within the higher education system for the first time. The intention was to produce nurses better able to meet the rapidly changing healthcare needs of society (UKCC, 1986).

The launch of the DipHE in 1989 in England and Wales, and in 1992 in Scotland, was undoubtedly a real victory. A framework, known as Project 2000, had been established for education and practice that produced not just safe nurses, but nurses who were able to improve the quality of patient care. Although Project 2000 was a great step forward, history never stands still, and evidence is accumulating that the Project 2000 reforms did not go far enough. Project 2000, like most policy decisions, is a compromise. James and Jones (1992) refer to compromise between political expediency, social conscience and professional interests. For example:

• Achieving student status was compromised by the requirement for 1000 hours of rostered service.

- The vast majority of Project 2000 students want to gain further qualifications – over half specifically refer to a degree as their goal.
- Students are forced into taking the hard road to a degree, either through part-time study or through another year of often self-funded study.

'Fitness for purpose'

The question of whether students are prepared to meet the demands of clinical practice at the point of registration has been debated under the phrase 'fitness for purpose'. A fundamental principle of pre-registration nurse education is thus the extent to which it provides new practitioners with an appropriate foundation for practice. However, although fitness for purpose may be the espoused objective of education programmes, the purpose is becoming increasingly difficult to define (Rushford and Ireland, 1997).

It is logical that the perspective of the Trusts as purchasers of education will reflect a predominantly local focus, and will not take account of characteristics such as epidemiological trends and current healthcare resources. The Trusts will also have a bias towards meeting short-term needs. Their purchase of education must, out of necessity, be based on a certain amount of means–end thinking; in other words, their ultimate goal is the selling of their services (Walters and Macleod Clark, 1993).

Such a model may have clear merit for the commissioning of post-registration education, which has the potential to be flexible and responsive in providing courses that meet local and short-term need. This has already been made evident by the range and diversity of courses that are offered by different educational providers, courses that reflect the local characteristics of the service units to which they have affiliation. However, this purchaser-led model may be fundamentally flawed for the provision of pre-registration education. By their very nature, these programmes are of a length and breadth that seeks to offer a comprehensive foundation for professional practice. Consequently, pre-registration education seeks to prepare nurses who are not only fit for purpose, but also equipped to practise within the rapidly changing world of healthcare (Rushford and Ireland, 1997).

Walters and Macleod Clark (1993) examined the perceptions of nurse managers with regard to contracting for pre-registration education. The comments of some respondents exemplify a utilitarian view of nurse education:

> I want a good quality, practical nurse at the end of training who is capable of taking responsibility.

> I want someone competent at a basic level from day one, not someone I have to train after registration, and a safe practitioner.

In contrast, nurse educators have concern for equipping the students to practise in a constantly and rapidly changing healthcare environment. In other words, they focus on the preparation of practitioners who are fit for the future. Thus their goals are focused far more on the educational process than the end product.

As Rushford and Ireland (1997) point out, in a contract-led climate, uncertainties inevitably exist in making decisions about how we prepare nurses who are best fit for purpose and fit for the future. This leads to tension between local and national perspectives, and between short-term and local needs. However, this does not need to be viewed as an 'either/or' situation. There must be recognition of the importance of equipping practitioners with a range of skills that have immediate currency at the point of registration. However, dominance must be given to the longer-term goals of the educational enterprise. Thus education must provide learners with a firm foundation on which, as life-long learners, they can continue to build throughout their professional careers.

Placement experience

Students now gain experience in a wide variety of care settings, spending less time in the hospital ward setting, where nurses have traditionally developed and practised their skills (Studdy *et al.*, 1994). The Diploma structure for nurse education has led to an increased emphasis on health promotion and the prevention of illness. There is therefore a focus on teaching nursing students from a 'wellness' model, thus limiting the students' experiences in the acute setting. However, many students, on qualifying, choose to work in an acute setting where patients are anything but 'well' and have complex needs. In 1998, the National Board for Nursing, Midwifery and Health Visting in Scotland noted widely expressed concerns that the practical skills of newly qualified nurses were less well developed than those of nurses trained prior to the advent of Project 2000 (NBS, 1998).

There has also been a dramatic increase in the time spent studying subjects such as psychology, sociology and health policy. This has, in turn, led to a significant reduction in the time that students spend acquiring psychomotor skills in the classroom. Consequently, a high proportion are expected to master what many would argue are essential nursing skills, such as hand-washing, bed-bathing, temperature, pulse and blood pressure monitoring, and numerous aseptic procedures, while on placement. Elkan and Robinson (1995), during their research into the implementation of the DipHE, found that students reported feeling awkward and ill at ease during their early ward placements. The students ascribed these feelings to a lack of practice competence.

Many employers, practitioners and students are becoming increasingly concerned that newly qualified pre-registration nurses are emerging from nursing programmes without essential clinical skills. In the report for the Department of Health (DoH) by the University of Warwick and Liverpool (Luker *et al.*, 1996), it was suggested that the practical skills exhibited by recently qualified nurses were found to be open to question and that nurses prepared by traditional methods were initially more competent practitioners. However, the new type of diploma programmes were producing nurses who were more confident, more theoretically knowledgeable and more able to judge when they needed supervision to perform clinical tasks. The report recommended that the National Health Service (NHS) and the Universities should work to improve collaboration between academic settings and the workplace to improve the understanding of, and provision for, the needs of the other. It was also argued that more attention should be paid to the teaching of practical skills during preparation, and to the provision of clinical support for newly qualified nurses. There are striking similarities between the findings of Luker *et al.* (1996) and the study by Runciman *et al.* (1998). The latter study suggests that newly qualified nurses need a considerable amount of help with practical skills and managerial and organisational skills. It recommends a carefully planned programme of skills development, moving from assisting students to gain confidence in use of equipment and techniques, towards progressive integration of knowledge with skilled performance in simulated and real situations.

Changing context of nurse education

The past few years, as outlined above, have been marked by far-reaching and rapid change in the environment within which the professional education of nurses takes place. The amalgamation of Colleges of Nursing and Midwifery and their subsequent transfer into higher education, together with the need for individuals to undertake degree or higher level study, has created a very stressful period for nurse lecturers. Crotty and Butterworth (1992) acknowledge the complexity of being required to be simultaneously a nurse, a teacher, a graduate in a specialist subject and both clinically and educationally credible. It is not surprising that, amidst these developments, the need for nurse lecturers to develop a role in the clinical area as the number of clinical teachers diminished, was afforded minimal importance by most nurse teachers and their managers (Wills, 1997).

This causes serious concern because, although the conflicts of meeting the demands of the clinical teaching role were documented in such a way as to lead to the recommendation to discontinue preparation for the role (Wright, 1984; Robertson, 1987; Martin, 1989; Clifford, 1993), there has been no apparent nationwide effort to provide the substitute for the aspects of the role that were positively rated. For example, Gott (1983) and Reid (1985) noted the positive benefits of the clinical teaching role in contributing towards a good learning environment. Moreover, the decision to discontinue the clinical teaching role was made against a background in which low priority was ascribed by nurse teachers to the clinical teaching role compared with the classroom role (Alexander, 1983; Jones, 1985). Luker *et al.* (1996) cited the importance of nurse lecturers' clinical competence and the challenge inherent in integrating the academic and practical. The need for strategies to ensure the clinical competence of nurse teachers has also been recommended (Luker *et al.*, 1996). Similarly, Phillips *et al.* (1996) stressed the need to be conscious of the need to make education clinically relevant and to provide appropriate clinical support structures. There is much to commend the preparation of doctors, in which the majority of teaching in the practice location is offered by clinically active experts.

Changing environment of practitioners

Several key national documents have outlined the changing context in which care is delivered, for example: *The National Health Service – A Service with Ambition* (DoH, 1996), *Challenges for Nursing and Midwifery Education in the Twenty-first Century – the Heathrow Debate* (DoH, 1994) and *A Vision for the Future – The Nursing, Midwifery and Health Visiting Contribution to Health and Healthcare* (DoH, 1993). These documents identify factors that have an influence on the types and numbers of practitioner needed, and on the knowledge, skills and attitudes they need in order to meet the health needs of the population. Far-reaching changes in both healthcare needs and service provision also make it increasingly difficult for student nurses to develop skills through repetition. These changes include a decline in the number of acute hospital beds, an increased emphasis upon day surgery and a move towards home care, coupled with a major shift of resources into community care provision. These factors have led to an increasingly finite, specialised, often unpredictable, clinical resource, with far sicker patients who should not be subjected to the practice of the novice (Studdy *et al.*, 1994).

The rapidly changing face of healthcare also means that technology is being introduced at an ever-increasing rate. The knowledge and competencies required by newly qualified nurses have therefore increased dramatically. Unfortunately, as noted above, the amount of time that student nurses spend in the clinical setting, where they can practise nursing skills, has not grown proportionately. On qualifying, nurses are faced with having to respond immediately to patients with unstable conditions and participate in decision-making that is often complicated by a shortened hospital stay. Qualified nurses are also becoming more specialised in given areas of practice and may themselves be struggling to keep up to date with new practices. Furthermore, as nursing roles change and expand, skills once regarded as 'extra' become core (Laurenson, 1997).

Consideration must also be given to the NHS reforms, which have resulted in clinical staff balancing conflicting demands in their management, clinical and educational roles (Jowett *et al.*, 1994). During recent years, many areas have seen a reduction in the number of permanent qualified staff, while the development of healthcare assistant training has meant an increased supervisory and assessment role. The qualified nurse's role, in terms of supervising Diploma students, has been reported to have been undermined by an inadequate initial preparation of trained staff. Service staff have also expressed concern about finding enough qualified staff to act as supervisors, the heavy burden of supervision given the student and staff numbers, and the heightened demands in terms of time and responsibility of teaching and supervising students undertaking the Common Foundation Programme (CFP) who possess not even basic practical nursing skills (Bedford *et al.*, 1993; Elkan and Robinson, 1995). Furthermore, according to feedback from students following clinical placements where teaching has occurred, it is questionable whether research-based practices are taught. Jowett *et al.* (1994), in a longitudinal study of the process of implementing Project 2000 programmes in 6 out of the 13 first-round demonstration districts, found that named mentors played a limited role in ensuring that a student's placement experiences were educationally sound. The increasingly busy clinical environment and the constantly changing student and staff population have led to a wide variation in the amount of time that clinicians are able to devote to teaching. Clinical staff also needed re-orientation towards the Diploma nurse's different profile of knowledge, skills, attitudes and confidence level.

Conclusion

The introduction of education-led Diploma programmes has been successful in increasing the academic status of nursing. However, higher cognitive skills, combined with more varied and less predictable clinical experience, have led to a perceived lack of skills and confidence. It is no longer sufficient to rely on students acquiring skills by unstructured exposure in the clinical placement. In light of experience with the DipHE, it is time to review the systems for skill acquisition and the role of the teacher in the practice placements.

Skills teaching must be structured and designed to prepare students for their placement experience so that they can optimise their learning within the context of increasingly scarce and finite resources. If the student's experience is not structured, students in the placement waste valuable clinical time learning how to perform skills rather than using that time to perfect skills and experience using them to care for real patients with real needs. In this way, students are able to gain most from their placement experience. The Clinical Skills Centre or Laboratory can be used for developing dexterity. This allows learning in clinical placements to concentrate on those skills that can only be learnt in the real care setting, such as interacting with a patient who is in pain. The use of a Skills Centre or Laboratory provides a suitable environment to learn the rudiments of a skill. In this way, learning opportunities can be structured and predictable, and the use of facilities can provide opportunities for consolidation and practice when not on placement.

References

Alexander, M (1983) *Learning to Nurse: Integrating Theory and Practice*. Edinburgh: Churchill Livingstone.

Bedford, H, Phillips, T, Robinson, J and Shostak, J (1993) *Assessing Competencies in Nursing and Midwifery Education*. London: English National Board.

Chapman, C (1980) The learner as worker: issues in nurse education. *Medical Teacher* **2**(5): 241–4.

Clifford, C (1993) The clinical role of the nurse teacher in the UK. *Journal of Advanced Nursing* 18(2): 281–9.

Crotty, M and Butterworth, T (1992) The emerging role of the nurse teacher in Project 2000 programmes in England, a literature review. *Journal of Advanced Nursing* 17: 1377–87.

Department of Health (1993) *A Vision for the Future – The Nursing, Midwifery and Health Visiting Contribution to Health and Healthcare*. London: HMSO.

Department of Health (1994) *Challenges for Nursing and Midwifery Education in the Twenty-first Century – the Heathrow Debate*. London: HMSO.

Department of Health (1996) *The National Health Service – A Service with Ambition*. London: HMSO.

Elkan, R and Robinson, J (1995) Project 2000: a review of published research. *Journal of Advanced Nursing* 22: 386–92.

Gomez, G E and Gomez, E A (1987) Learning of psychomotor skills: laboratory versus patient care setting. *Journal of Nursing Education* 26(1): 20–4.

Gott, M (1983) The preparation of the student for learning in the clinical setting. In Davies, B D (ed.) *Research into Nurse Education*. Beckenham: Croom Helm.

Greenwood, J (1993) Reflective practice: a critique of the work of Argyris and Schön. *Journal of Advanced Nursing* 18: 1183–7.

James, J and Jones, D (1992) Education for the future: meeting changing needs. In Slevin, V and Buckenham, M (eds) *Project 2000: The Teachers Speak*. Edinburgh: Campus Press.

Jones, J A (1985) A study of nurse tutors' conceptualisation of their ward teaching role. *Journal of Advanced Nursing* 10: 349–60.

Jowett, S, Walton, I and Payne, S (1994) *Challenges and Change in Nurse Education: A Study of the Implementation of Project 2000*. Slough: NFER.

Knowles, M (1990) *The Adult Learner: The Neglected Species*. Huston: Gulf.

Laurenson, S (1997) Changing roles of nurses in Scotland: a survey of developing clinical roles within the NHS trusts in Scotland. *Health Bulletin* 55(5): 331–8.

Levin, P (1998) Divided they surely fall. *Times Higher Education Supplement*, February 6, p. 28.

Luker, K, Carlisle, C and Kirk, S (1993) *The Evolving Role of the Nurse Teacher in the Light of Educational Reforms*. London: ENB.

Luker, K, Carlisle, C, Riley, E, Stilwell, J, Davies, C and Wilson, R (1996) *Project 2000 Fitness for Purpose: Report to the Department of Health*. The University of Liverpool and the University of Warwick.

Martin, L (1989) *Clinical Education in Perspective*. London: RCN.

National Board for Nursing, Midwifery and Health Visiting for Scotland (1998) *Information Base on Arrangements which Support the Development of Clinical Practice in Pre-Registration Nursing Programmes in Scotland*. Edinburgh: NBS.

Orton, H D (1981) *Ward Learning Climate: A Study of the Role of the Ward Sister in Relation to Student Nurse Learning on the Ward*. London: RCN.

Phillips, T, Bedford, H, Robinson J and Schostak L (1994) *Education, Dialogue and Assessment: Creating Partnerships for Improving Practice*. London: ENB.

Reid, N G (1985) *Wards in Chancery*. London: RCN.

Robertson, C M (1987) *A Very Special Form of Teaching*. London: RCN.

Ruciman, P, Dewar, B and Goulbourne A (1998) *Project 2000 in Scotland: Employers' Needs and the Skills of Newly Qualified Project 2000 Staff Nurses*. Edinburgh; National Board for Nursing, Midwifery and Health Visting for Scotland.

Rushford, H and Ireland, L (1997) Fit for purpose? The contextual forces underpinning the provision of nurse education in the UK. *Nurse Education Today* **17**: 437–41.

Studdy, S J, Nicol, M and Fox-Hiley, A (1994) Teaching and learning clinical skills. Part 2: Development of a teaching model and schedule of skills development. *Nurse Education Today* **14**: 186–93.

United Kingdom Central Council for Nursing, Midwifery and Health Visiting (1986) *Project 2000: A New Preparation for Practice*. London: UKCC.

Walters, G and Macleod Clark, J (1993) Nurse manager's perceptions of contracting for education, Part 1. *Nurse Education Today* **13**: 401–8.

Wills, M E (1997) Link teachers behaviours: student nurses' perceptions. *Nurse Education Today* **17**: 232–46.

Wright, S (1984) Piggy in the middle. *Senior Nurse* **1**: 11.

2

Is Simulation the Answer?

Maggie Nicol

Introduction

The introduction of Project 2000 curricula (UKCC, 1986) has meant that students of nursing now spend less time (40 per cent of the total as opposed to 60 per cent pre-Project 2000) in a much wider variety of hospital- and community-based clinical placements. As Neary (1997) comments, the practical experience now extends into 'homes, schools, factories, shops and every community agency even remotely connected to healthcare delivery' (1997: 46). This, and the large number of students in each cohort to be accommodated, means that students spend less time on placement in hospital wards, where nurses have traditionally learnt or refined most of their clinical skills.

In the past, student nurses were introduced to a variety of clinical skills in the practical room of the School of Nursing. Here the skills were demonstrated by a tutor and then practised by the students to ensure that they had some notion of how to perform a range of 'basic' procedures before contact with real patients and clients. However, Schools of Nursing were usually situated close to a hospital, which meant that the teaching was able to continue into the real setting. A tutor, accompanied by a group of new recruits, would visit a ward to demonstrate some fundamental nursing skill such as a bed bath or wound dressing on a real patient.

13

The 1970s saw a move away from the use of practical rooms. Their use was considered undesirable because they created an artificial situation that bore no resemblance to the real care setting. In addition, equipment and tutors were often out of date, which only served to widen the theory–practice gap between what was taught in school and what was current practice in the placements. The only place to learn clinical skills, it was argued, was in the real care setting under the direction and supervision of staff who were clinically competent. Such an approach was later supported by Gomez and Gomez (1987), who demonstrated that students learning in the real care setting gained competence and confidence more quickly than those confined to the Skills Laboratory. However, as discussed .in Chapter 1, learning in the real care setting requires one-to-one teaching and supervision, and the pressures currently experienced by qualified nurses in the clinical areas mean that this is often not possible. Practitioners are faced with having to balance the demands of increasingly dependent patients with the educational needs of the students (While, 1991). In addition, the large cohorts of students now being recruited mean that clinical staff may well have to take responsibility for several students at one time (Clifford, 1994). Although many nurse lecturers provide clinical teaching for students, this usually only amounts to a few hours per student per placement, so the majority of the teaching and supervision has to be provided by the clinical staff.

All of these factors have contributed to criticisms of Project 2000 courses, not least by the students themselves, for being too focused on the sociocultural aspects of health and illness, at the expense of clinical skills (Neary, 1997). This has led Schools of Nursing to re-examine the ways in which clinical skills are developed. The challenge of finding sufficient, quality clinical experiences has long been a problem facing nurse educators in the United States, where student numbers are great and clinical facilities overcrowded (Whitis, 1985). Although desirable and, with one-to-one teaching and supervision arguably the best way to learn, it is no longer possible to rely solely on students learning in the clinical placements. The purpose of this chapter is to discuss the use of simulation as an adjunct to clinical placements as a means of acquiring clinical skills.

What is simulation?

There is a wealth of literature on the use of simulation with a variety of different professional and occupational groups. However, on examination, much of the literature refers to simulation *games*. These games, ranging from simple board games or role play at one end to virtual reality at the other, are designed to increase social and professional skills such as communication, problem-solving, leadership and decision-making. Such tools have been used in nursing and are useful tools for the development of problem-solving and clinical management skills (Wildman and Reeves, 1996). However, they are not designed to encourage the development of practical clinical skills.

In this chapter, the term 'simulation' refers to the use of simulated settings to create a realistic replication of the real world. Gohring (1979) defined simulation as 'created experiences that simplify reality which cannot or should not be experienced first-hand by a student because of inexperience, complexity, danger, cost or other reasons' (cited by Whitis, 1985: 161). The use of simulation means that the real world can be created without all the disadvantages, such as real clinical demands and emergency situations. Whitis (1985), in a review of the use of simulation in nurse education in the USA, concluded that it was 'a more efficient and safer method of providing clinical experiences' (1985: 163). There is comparatively little literature reporting the use of simulated settings as a means of teaching clinical skills. What there is tends to favour the use of simulation, but there is as yet no conclusive evidence that its use improves clinical practice (Roberts *et al.*, 1992). Whitis (1985) suggested that there was some evidence that the use of clinical simulation in medical education was more effective than instruction with real patients; however, this, has not been confirmed by other studies.

Advantages of simulation

Safe learning environment

One of the major concerns of students nurses is the fear of doing harm to patients (Neary, 1997). Many student nurses find the busy hospital ward a bewildering setting in which to learn new skills. Acute care settings, which are where students will find most opportunities to learn and practise their clinical skills, are becoming increasingly complex. Patients are in hospital for shorter periods and are more vulnerable to care by an inexperienced student. Factors such as patient safety, comfort and the right to privacy all influence the student's learning (Whitis, 1985). Also, clinical placements include many community-based experiences, where the opportunities to practise fundamental nursing skills on a regular basis to develop mastery are minimal. The simulated care setting provides a safe environment in which to learn and refine clinical skills, safe in the knowledge that mistakes do not matter and no harm will come to the patient. By lowering the level of anxiety of both students and teachers, more knowledge can be acquired in a shorter period of time (Dahl, 1984).

Controlled learning environment

Another advantage of the use of simulation is that the simulated clinical experience can be controlled according to the level of skill and learning needs of the students. In the simulated setting, patients and clients will react and respond in a predictable way in order to provide the students with the appropriate learning. Thus, unless it is appropriate to the students' learning outcomes, the patient will not suddenly collapse, have an epileptic fit or refuse all treatment, as can happen in the real care setting. This results in more predictable learning. Dahl (1984) argued that because the use of simulation is exciting, fun and ultimately 'real' for the student, the retention of information is greater.

Bridging the theory–practice gap

The use of simulation means that many different simulated settings can be created in one location. For example, community settings, such as a patient's home or practice nurse's clinic, can be created alongside a hospital ward, out-patients department, accident and emergency department, children's ward or maternity department. Now that most Schools of Nursing and Midwifery are incorporated into Universities, they are often situated on large campuses a good distance from many of the clinical placements. The provision of a skills-teaching facility on campus makes it possible to teach clinical skills at the appropriate point in the curriculum, thus linking theory and practice. If students have to rely solely on clinical placements to develop their clinical skills, many opportunities for making links between the theory, for example the principles of asepsis, and the practical skill of performing a wound dressing, will be lost. Relying entirely on the clinical placements can mean that the development of clinical skills is *ad hoc* and dependent on what a particular placement has to offer. The use of simulation enables clinical skills to be clearly defined as learning outcomes for each part of the programme.

Experiential learning

Simulated settings offer the additional advantage that nursing students act as patients for their colleagues when learning to perform the various skills. This means that they not only learn how to perform the skill and increase their dexterity, but also experience how it feels to be fed by someone else, to be lifted in a mechanical hoist or to have a blood pressure cuff inflated to 250 mmHg! Such learning experiences, which provide such valuable insights into the patient's world, cannot be provided in the real care setting.

Economic considerations

Nursing is a practice-based profession, so it is vital that the clinical skills that are the 'tools of the trade' are given the same emphasis as all the other disciplines, such as psychology, biology and sociology. Clinical placements no longer form the largest part of the 3-year programme, so it is vital that clinical skills are given timetable time and are assessed in the same way as other subjects in the curriculum. If simulation is not used, nurse educators must accompany students to the clinical areas in order to demonstrate essential nursing skills such as meeting hygiene needs, caring for a patient with a chest drain or performing a 12-lead ECG. This can mean travelling considerable distances, and as only small groups can be accommodated, a teacher:student ratio of around 1:4 or 1:6 is all that is usually possible. It also relies on there being a suitable patient or client available at the appropriate time who consents to being observed by a number of student nurses.

The use of simulation enables larger groups of students (up to 20) to observe a realistic demonstration set in the holistic context of a patient scenario. Students can ask questions at any time, and the demonstration can be repeated as many times as necessary. The use of simulation also has the advantage that students can be encouraged to discuss the situation and make links between theory and practice in a way that may well not be possible or desirable with a real patient. For example, if teaching post-operative observations, to discuss the signs of haemorrhage in front of the patient might cause anxiety or distress. Also, aspects of care that might cause embarrassment in real practice, such as washing the genital area of a patient of the opposite sex, can openly be discussed and ideas generated on how to deal with such situations when they occur. Students working together have been shown to learn more effectively because they observe each other and discuss decisions and priorities (Neary, 1997).

Learning can be fun

Learning to care in a busy clinical area can be bewildering and nerve-wracking, and students have identified a fear of harming patients as a major source of anxiety (Neary, 1997). Making a mistake can provide a very negative learning experience and may lead to a loss of confidence. Learning in the simulated setting, on the other hand, can be fun as well as educational. As long as there is an adequate level of supervision, mistakes can be used to provide valuable learning opportunities for the whole group. The use of video feedback further enhances the learning by enabling students to gain insight into their abilities and to identify their own strengths and weaknesses. The use of simulation means that students can become dextrous in a variety of essential nursing skills before being required to perform them on real patients.

Assessment of competence

A simulated setting can provide a realistic environment for the assessment of clinical skills, but one in which the complexity and other variables are controlled. Also, if nurse educators are directly involved in the assessment of clinical competence, they are required to define elements of the skill and assessment criteria. As Kolb and Shugart (1984) have pointed out, this means that faculty are 'forced to provide a specific means of evaluating objectives which may have been skimmed over previously' (1984: 85). The assessment of competence by the Objective Structured Clinical Examination (OSCE) (Harden and Gleeson, 1979), in which students are required to perform a number of skills in a simulated care setting and are assessed by lecturers using detailed checklists, is discussed further in Chapters 3 and 4.

Self-directed learning

Students are increasingly being encouraged to take responsibility for their own learning and to develop the skills to become life-long learners. With their academic studies, this is relatively easy to achieve, but when developing clinical skills, it is not so simple. Students are not able to negotiate extra time in a clinical placement in the same way as they can arrange extra tutorials or spend more time in the library for their academic work. The use of simulation means that students are able to spend as much time as they need in order to achieve dexterity in a skill. It also means that they can maintain their skills during periods between clinical placements and 'revise' them prior to clinical assessments.

Disadvantages of simulation

Resources

The provision of a modern skills-teaching facility requires the commitment of a considerable amount of resources, financial and human, if it is not to suffer from the same criticisms as the old practical rooms. Financial considerations include the provision of a sufficiently large and flexible teaching facility, fully equipped with models, simulators and up-to-date equipment such as that encountered in any real clinical setting. The capital costs incurred when setting up such a facility are considerable, but so too are the running costs. It is important that the realism is such that single-use items such as syringes and needles are not re-used in the interests of economy. The students may not realise that re-use is only acceptable in the simulated setting and may do the same in practice. Therefore teaching large groups of students skills such as injections involves equally large numbers of syringes, needles and swabs and so on.

Teaching within such a facility is labour intensive as, in order to facilitate and supervise practice, groups of no more than 20 can usually be accommodated. In addition, because of the nature of some of the skills being taught and the amount of supervision required (for example, moving and handling), two or even three teachers will be required to ensure safety. In addition to teaching, human resources are also needed to manage the facility, organise room bookings, order stocks and so on.

Clinical competence of lecturers

In order to be able to teach clinical skills, lecturers need to be clinically competent themselves. While most Schools of Nursing and Midwifery have a system whereby all lecturers are required to maintain links with clinical practice areas, not all lecturers practise regularly, so would not consider themselves sufficiently up to date to teach clinical skills. This means that either the responsibility for skills teaching falls on a small group of lecturers who are clinically competent, who have to repeat themselves several times a week to the small groups, or on lecturers who are not clinically competent. If their skills are not up to date such lecturers quickly lose credibility with students and clinical practitioners alike.

Requiring all lecturers to maintain their clinical competence may be laudable, but it is often difficult to achieve given the increasing academic workload and the geographical distance involved in getting to many clinical areas. Trying to meet the demands to be a teacher, assessor/marker, researcher and clinical practitioner may be too much for many lecturers.

Transfer of skills

One of the advantages of simulation is that real-life situations can be created without all the distractions and inconveniences of real life. However, this can also be perceived as a disadvantage. Those who oppose the use of simulation argue that, like the old practical rooms, Skills Laboratories merely create a false situation that fails to teach students about real-life clinical situations. Nor is there any proof that it helps them to transfer skills learnt using simulation into their clinical placements (Neary, 1994). Although a study in the 1970s found that the use of flight simulators promoted both the achievement and maintenance of performance in actual flying (Cream *et al.*, 1978, cited by Hegstad and Zsohar, 1986), the realism created by flight simulators is far superior to that achieved in most nursing skills laboratories.

Conclusion

If one subscribes to the belief that clinical practice is central to nursing, the development of the clinical 'tools' of practice must be considered to be equally as important as the cognitive skills required. In order to reflect that belief, curriculum time must be devoted to clinical skills acquisition. The development of clinical skills cannot be left to chance to be acquired in an *ad hoc* fashion in the clinical placements. The responsibility for ensuring that students develop the skills they need to become autonomous practitioners cannot be left to the students themselves or to the clinical practitioners. Clinical practitioners clearly have a vital role to play in the development of future nurses, but just as nurse educators would presumably not rely on their clinical colleagues to provide the sociology, psychology and biology components of the course, neither should they be expected to be solely responsible for the clinical aspects. The role of clinical practitioners, particularly in pre-registration programmes, is one of supervision of the students as they practise and refine their skills. The teaching of fundamental clinical skills must remain the responsibility of nurse educators. To do otherwise would mean that the need to have nurses teaching nursing could rightly be challenged.

The use of simulation provides a way of accomplishing this in an economical way. It gives students a safe environment in which to practise the skills they need and provides opportunities for them to arrange additional practice with skills they find difficult, thus making them responsible for their own development. The use of simulation will never replace the need for quality, well-supervised clinical placements, but, as Gohring (1979) has pointed out, simulation allows for the creation of situations that 'cannot or should not' be experienced first hand by students. Patients and clients have a right to expect skilled nursing care and, it could be argued, should not be used as 'audiovisual aids' to enable student learning.

Used creatively by clinically competent nurse lecturers, simulation can provide an important foundation and enable students to develop a sufficient level of skill to make the most of the valuable learning experiences that only real patients and clients in real care settings can provide. However, the use of simulation must never be seen as a replacement for clinical placements. It must be viewed as part of the whole clinical learning experience, a part that provides opportunities to achieve specific learning outcomes that may not be possible, desirable or likely to be achieved in the real care setting.

References

Clifford, C (1994) Assessment of clinical practice and the role of the nurse teacher. *Nurse Education Today* **14**: 272–9.

Cream, B W, Eggemeier, F T and Klein, G (1978) A strategy for the development of training devices. *Human Factors* **20**: 145–58.

Dahl, J (1984) Structured experience: a risk free approach to reality-based learning. *Journal of Nursing Education* **23**(1): 34–7.

Gohring, R J (1979) All in the game. *Discovery* **3**: 20–3.

Gomez, G E and Gomez, E A (1987) Learning of psychomotor skills: laboratory versus patient care setting. *Journal of Nursing Education* **26**(1): 20–4.

Harden, R and Gleeson, F (1979) Assessment of clinical competence using an objective structured clinical examination (OSCE). *Medical Education* **13**: 41–51.

Hegstad, L N and Zsohar, H (1986) A study of the cost effectiveness of providing psychomotor practice in teaching intravenous infusion techniques. *Journal of Nursing Education* **25**(1): 10–14.

Kolb, S E and Shugart, E B (1984) Evaluation: is simulation the answer? *Journal of Nursing Education*, **23**(2): 84–6.

Neary, M (1994) Teaching practical skills in colleges. *Nursing Standard*, **8**(27): 35–8.

Neary, M (1997) Project 2000 students' survival kit: a return to the practical room (nursing skills laboratory). *Nurse Education Today* **17**: 46–52.

Roberts, J, While, A and Fitzpatrick, M (1992) Simulation: current status in nurse education. *Nurse Education Today* **12**: 409–15.

United Kingdom Central Council for Nursing, Midwifery and Health Visiting (1986) *Project 2000: A New Preparation for Practice*. London: UKCC.

While, A (1991) The problem of clinical evaluation – a review. *Nurse Education Today* **11**: 448–53.

Whitis, G (1985) Simulation in teaching clinical nursing. *Journal of Nursing Education* **24**(4): 161–3.

Wildman, S and Reeves, M (1996) The utilisation and evaluation of a simulation game in pre-registration nurse education. *Nurse Education Today* **16**: 334–9.

3

Development of a Skills Centre

Beryl Howard

Introduction

The establishment of the Skills Centre in the Department of Nursing at the University of Salford has been, without question, one of the greatest challenges faced by the department. This chapter will describe the history and the reasons for the Centre's development. The important issue of funding will be discussed, along with the identification of the key players and the role of the NHS Trusts. The teaching, learning and assessment methods used will be described, and the chapter will conclude with an overview of future planned developments.

Context

This is not a book about the history of nurse education, but the impact of the merger of established Schools of Nursing and their subsequent integration into higher education on the establishment of the Skills Centre has been quite significant. It is therefore necessary to provide an overview of the local developments and their influence. These are by no means unique, and many readers are likely to have had similar experiences. In April 1990, three Schools of Nursing merged to form the West Pennine College of Health Studies, in line with the national strategy to streamline nurse education. At this time, nurse teachers within the newly formed college had not been exposed to Project 2000 (UKCC, 1986), which was still in its embryonic phase, and were largely 'General' nurse teachers, that is, those teachers who would teach 'Adult Nursing' when eventually involved with Project 2000 programme. On the other side of Manchester, two other Schools of Nursing had recently merged and had commenced the Diploma in Professional Studies (Project 2000) course in October 1990. During the validation and implementation process, strong links with the University of Salford had been developed, which meant that the teaching staff had experience of working with higher education and the process of accreditation. In 1994, the two Colleges merged to form the Northern College of Nursing, Midwifery and Health Studies, and in April 1996 became the largest department in the University of Salford.

Introduction of skills teaching into the curriculum

As the integration was completed, the Project 2000 curriculum became the only curriculum. Teachers were expected quickly to adapt to and implement a curriculum that they had not developed, so did not feel 'ownership' of. This inevitably led to a number of tensions because of different ideologies. One major area of concern was the lack of clinical skills teaching. The curriculum document specified clinical skills teaching, but when this was translated into a timetable, it became, for example, the taking and recording of blood pressure for groups of 70 students in a lecture theatre. This was due partly to the lack of facilities to accommodate large groups, and partly to the belief in nursing at the time that clinical skills were best learnt in the real practice setting. Such an approach seemed logical and was supported by research (Gomez and Gomez, 1987), but it failed to acknowledge the realities of an over-stretched health service in which increasing workloads and reducing numbers of qualified staff often resulted in unpredictable teaching and supervision (Studdy *et al.*, 1994).

At the same time, the development of Regional Purchasing Consortia and the growing requirement to be 'contract aware' meant that educational institutions had a greater reason to clarify what clinical skills future employers required of nurses. In discussions with a number of executive nurses and nurse managers from local Trusts, it emerged that many felt that junior students were ill prepared for their clinical experiences and were consequently unable to contribute to the delivery of patient care. Clinical staff and managers appeared to be more than satisfied with the cognitive abilities of students, especially their reflective and reasoning capabilities, but comments related to the lack of skills acquisition were certainly borne out in early evaluations of Project 2000 (Elkan and Robinson, 1991).

Personal experience as a clinical teacher supported the view that clinical staff have insufficient time to teach the very fundamentals of clinical skills to students who have received no prior tuition. A review of the literature supported this and subscribed to the need for skills teaching within Project 2000 courses (Jowett *et al.*, 1994; Studdy *et al.*, 1994).

Key staff

A small working group of seven eager volunteers was established. Over a 2-month period, four of the volunteers visited St Bartholomew's School of Nursing, London, where a Clinical Skills Centre and programme for skills teaching had been established (Studdy *et al.*, 1994). The facilities were excellent and provided ideas for our own development. The visits also enabled discussion about how others had persuaded their colleagues of the value of skills teaching. The suggestion by the working group that we should consider introducing skills workshops into the programme delighted some members of staff, but others were dismayed. They were particularly concerned that re-introducing the old practical room was a retrograde step.

The well-documented issues of practical rooms and their demise was discussed (Neary, 1994). It was evident that a great deal of effort would be required to ensure that any new facility was not only equipped with modern equipment, as found in clinical areas, but also appropriately staffed and maintained. In addition, there was a need to assess the clinical competence of teaching staff, some of whom openly admitted that they considered themselves to be 'out of date' in terms of clinical skills. Discussions also focused on *what* to teach and when. The curriculum was so congested that there was no space in it to facilitate extra sessions, so the teaching of practical skills would have to be undertaken in the students' self-directed study periods until such time as the curriculum was re-validated. A further consideration was the larger and ever-increasing student numbers. In order to achieve manageably sized groups for skills teaching, the cohorts would have to be subdivided. These smaller workshop groups would then be timetabled to attend the college in their self-directed study time. The majority of students accepted the change as a positive development, although a very small minority felt the change to be intrusive on their study time, time which in some cases was spent undertaking work to supplement their bursaries.

It was decided to pilot the skills workshops for a period of 4 months and to evaluate their influence in terms of, first, the students' perception of their effectiveness in the clinical area, and second, the clinical staff's perception of the students' contribution to care delivery. The choice of pilot sites was dictated by those which still had practical rooms containing an appropriate amount of equipment. The pilot period in fact continued for 6 months because the evaluation took longer to organise than had at first been anticipated. The data resulting from a short questionnaire, along with anecdotal evidence gained from discussions between clinical staff and link teachers, demonstrated how positively the workshops were viewed. The positive evaluations served to encourage those who were actively involved and quietly stimulated the interest of the less enthusiastic teachers, some of whom were continuing to express negative views.

There was a growing demand to explore the area of skills acquisition in nursing students and other professions allied to medicine, and in November 1995, the Department of Nursing hosted a Multidisciplinary Skills Conference. Ninety delegates attended and speakers included those with experience in the area of skills acquisition and skills teaching from a variety of professions, including nursing, medicine, physiotherapy and occupational therapy. Networking, both during and following the conference, was very encouraging and provided the stimulus to continue with the project's development. The working group continued to meet regularly and produced a review paper that was to inform the college management team of the effectiveness of the skills workshops and to seek funding to develop a Skills Centre.

Practical room recycled?

The proposal to establish a 'Skills Centre' within the main College campus was met with a degree of scepticism as the memory of run-down practical rooms was still fresh. It was vital that it was sited on the main campus site because the peripheral sites would eventually close as the merger into higher education took place. Eventually, after lengthy discussion, the sum of £20,000 from the non-pay budget lines was made available, providing a suitable room could be identified. That was no easy task as most of the teaching accommodation was at near maximum usage. The possibility of developing a Skills Centre in a closed ward was explored but reluctantly rejected as it became apparent that the ward could not be adequately secured and that equipment would undoubtedly be removed to supplement ward stocks. A further problem was that of cleaning. The School would be required to pay the Trust for domestic services, and it was felt that this would be an unacceptable drain on resources.

Another avenue explored was the possibility of sharing a new building at the hospital, which was to house a Skills Laboratory for use by medical students. The Post-graduate Medical Dean was approached about possible collaboration in skills teaching, and although he was initially keen on a joint venture with the Department, the huge numbers of potential nursing students prompted the Dean reluctantly to decline to co-operate in the project. Thus a decision was taken to develop the teaching facility on the main campus site.

Resourcing issues

The identified room required a major overhaul in terms of decoration and the fitting of storage cupboards and a sink unit with elbow taps. Only one storage room, off the main room, was available to us. This was to prove to be a significant problem as the equipment levels increased. Hospital supplies departments were extremely helpful in assisting with the purchasing of clinical equipment, for example beds, lockers, bed tables and intravenous infusion stands. Catalogues were obtained and the majority of the £20,000 that had been made available was very quickly spent. It was important that the refurbishment was completed quickly because students at the main campus were being taught clinical skills in very inferior settings while it was being developed.

As the Skills Centre began to take shape, and it became apparent that there was a real commitment and that developments were more co-ordinated, more and more teachers became interested in the teaching of clinical skills. The Skills Working Group began to grow (the membership at this stage being around 25), and there were difficulties managing such a large number of staff. However, it was important not to turn anyone away as the number of students using the Skills Centre would require either input from someone on a full-time basis or the assurance that a large number of teachers were available to deliver the sessions.

As anticipated, 12 months after the commencement of the pilot study, 2 out of the 3 peripheral sites closed, and most of the teaching of clinical skills was concentrated at the main campus. One practical site remained on the only other remote campus, and the availability of this facility was to become important as time passed.

Teaching and learning strategies

Third-year students, who had not been viewed as a priority group because of their previous exposure to practice, wrote expressing their 'growing concern regarding the lack of practical skills gained during the Common Foundation

Programme'. They realised that many skills would be gained when on 'rostered duty' but felt that 'this time will be more advantageous if a basic grounding in nursing techniques was gained prior to this time'. This letter, received during the evaluative phase, acted as a stimulus to continue. The students' programme leader was contacted, and specific arrangements were made to schedule them into the Skills Centre at the earliest opportunity. The students had, by this stage of their educational development, been exposed to and participated in many nursing skills, so had had the opportunity to reflect on underlying principles and be introduced to the more technical skills such as catheterisation.

Scheduling of the skills workshops during the CFP was dominated by the need to accommodate the huge number of students within the limited facilities available. The facilities could physically only accommodate a maximum of 20 students. These workshops were linked to clinical practice experience, and account was taken of the students' stage of training or level of clinical experience. Interpersonal skills development was viewed as an integral part of the workshops. The teaching of interpersonal skills was to be an ongoing issue during the early planning stage as those teachers with a specific interest in this particular area, largely mental health teachers, were concerned that the skills workshops would concentrate too heavily on psychomotor skills, to the detriment of psychological and interpersonal considerations. It was suggested that those teachers assist with the teaching of skills in order to ensure that their concerns did not materialise. However, like many nurse teachers, they felt concerned that they no longer possessed the necessary skills to teach psychomotor skills to students. Although most teachers had a practice link role, this often did not involve actual hands-on care. This was to prove to be a pivotal issue in the development of a core group of teachers who would be responsible for skills teaching.

Staff development

As more and more teachers acknowledged the value of teaching clinical skills, this acted as a catalyst to determine what was 'current practice' and stimulated some staff who had previously only been involved in educational audit activities to become involved in practice in order to develop their skills. However, not all staff recognised the need to update their clinical skills, and this remains a cause of some concern within the department. Where it was felt appropriate, company representatives and clinical nurse specialists were invited to our meetings to discuss current equipment and its use in order to promote the development of the lecturer's practical skills.

Integration and scheduling of the workshops into the curriculum

During the first 12 months of the project, students were taught skills based around the 'activities of living'. The philosophy of the Skills Centre was that we would concentrate on developing fundamental, but nevertheless essential, skills in our students. During the CFP, they were taught skills related to eating and drinking, mobility (the statutory moving and handling), personal cleansing and dressing, including bed-making and patient comfort, elimination and so on. A further £7000 was provided to purchase further equipment as necessary, but as this was a relatively small sum and we were developing the facility from nothing, there was a need in the early days to procure disposable equipment from the clinical areas. This practice became more and more difficult as ward managers had to be mindful of their budgets. Eventually, a recurrent budget to purchase disposables was established, an acknowledgement that at last the value of the skills workshops had been recognised.

The development of a new pre-registration Diploma in Nursing enabled us to integrate skills workshops into the programme. No longer were they to be viewed as an 'add on' to a nurse education course: clinical skills were given the status that they undoubtedly deserved.

Because of the huge increase in student numbers, the workshops continue to be an immense demand on human resources. Cohorts of up to 250 students had to be subdivided into 14 workshop groups in order to facilitate effective teaching. Each of the 14 groups had three full-day workshops in semester I, two full-day workshops in semesters II and III, and one full-day workshop in semester IV. Each workshop had its own schedule, and this meant that a teacher could be required to teach the same skill 14 times over a 7-week period. There was occasionally a tension between staffing the skills workshops and other aspects of the course. As further cohorts joined the Department of Nursing, the demand on human and other resources intensified. In January 1997, a second room became available, which was developed as a 'moving and handling' facility. Again from the non-pay budget, £8000 was made available to purchase equipment specific for the purpose.

The first session of the first workshop is related to the Skills Centre philosophy and ground rules, which were felt necessary in order to guide students through the Centre safely. The 'rules' concern safety issues, punctuality, confidentiality and professionalism.

Students are encouraged to be sensitive towards their colleagues if mistakes are made, for example, or if concerns and fears are expressed. The principal purpose of the workshops is that the students can learn the 'art' and 'craft' of nursing in a safe environment where they can make mistakes without fear of harming a patient or client and without fear of ridicule. As the students progress through the workshops, the skills become increasingly demanding. First aid and cardio-pulmonary resuscitation skills (the basics of which are taught in semester I) continue to be developed in semesters II and III. The care of patients who are dying and their families is also explored in semester III, as are neurological observations and their meaning.

During the first three semesters, students are exposed to and practise those essential nursing skills in which they, as junior students, can be expected to participate. The workshop scheduled to take place in semester IV (commencing at week 60 of the course) is devoted to the formative evaluation of those skills.

It is recognised that not all skills can be taught in the Skills Centre. In some areas, for example orthopaedics, it is not possible to provide the necessary equipment or clinical expertise within the Skills Centre. In these circumstances, the principles are taught and the students are then required, during an appropriate placement and through a 'learning contract', to develop the appropriate skills.

Assessment of competence – Objective Structured Clinical Examination (OSCE)

Studdy *et al.* (1994) describe the value of formatively assessing students' progress in the area of skills acquisition. A programme of OSCEs was developed by a subgroup of the Skills Working Group and used to evaluate the development of skills in the Diploma in Nursing programme. As the new cohort required the main Skills Centre facility for semester I workshops, the only other skills teaching facility sited on a peripheral campus was used for the OSCEs. A 3-week period was identified, and the course leader for the semester IV students allocated pairs of students each hour of the 8-hour day, 5 days a week for 3 weeks. Dictated largely by the size of the room to be used and also by the staffing implications, two workstations were provided, each fully equipped with beds, lockers, patient chairs and so on. Other equipment was provided on nearby tables or trolleys. Full hand-washing facilities were also available. Junior students were asked to volunteer to act as the two 'patients' needed per day.

Members of the subgroup developed scenarios within which the students were asked to provide 'essential' care. The two scenarios, which the students were given 3 weeks prior to their evaluations, while portraying completely different situations, required similar skills to be performed. The common elements were that the student was required to take and record the 'patient's' temperature, pulse, respiration and blood pressure, and use moving and handling techniques. The differences were that one scenario required the student to seek to obtain a sample of urine, whereas the other required the student to wash the hands and face of the 'patient'. The group also developed associated critique sheets, which were to be used at the time of evaluation in order to maintain as much objectivity and consistency as possible. Feedback was given to the student using the critique sheet immediately following the evaluation, and the feedback was then kept in the student's Portfolio following discussion with his or her personal teacher. Each workstation had an 'evaluator', a lecturer who was involved with the teaching of clinical skills.

Benefits of the OSCE

It was believed that this formative evaluation would be of benefit to the students who are assessed summatively in the clinical area for the first time later in the same semester. The areas of role responsibility, interpersonal skills, caring skills and clinical skills are summatively assessed in practice. Preliminary evaluation of the OSCEs suggests that they have proved to be extremely beneficial not only to the students, but also to the 'patients' and the evaluators, as described below.

Students

While the students felt apprehensive in their anticipation of the OSCEs, the majority of them (82 per cent) felt that the immediate feedback given to them was invaluable. However, a small minority (16 per cent) felt that the distance that they had to travel for the short period of time outweighed any benefits gained.

'Patients'

The 'patients' were junior students (see above). Without fail, all of those students involved in the role play found the experience to be of great value, as suggested by O'Neill and McCall (1996). As expected, some gained more than others, if only through the interaction with students and evaluators.

Evaluators

The OSCEs have been extremely expensive in terms of human resources. It was also necessary to draw up reserve lists of 'patients' and 'evaluators' who could be called upon at short notice in case of sickness. Without exception, those teachers involved found the experience tiring but extremely informative.

Two major issues emerged that need to be addressed. The first is that the students find the workshops invaluable but feel that more time is required for practice. Second, it would appear that too much time is being spent on the theory underpinning skills as opposed to the actual hands-on practice. Cognisance will be taken of these valuable comments when planning the workshops for future groups. The value gained from organising and facilitating the OSCEs was well worth the effort.

Future developments

There are a number of issues/developments that require consideration if the skills workshops that have become so integral to our educational philosophy are to be improved.

Resources

There are currently at least 20 lecturers who facilitate the workshops. Because we admit such large numbers of students and have to utilise a 'rolling programme' of workshops, knowing that this huge resource is available is comforting. However, the appointment of two clinical lecturer–practitioners whose sole responsibility will be to teach skills, albeit supported by a core group of lecturers, is currently being considered. The appointment of these staff would ensure greater consistency and continuity. The establishment of a manageable system of ordering equipment, particularly disposable equipment, has proved to be the only major problem area. Ordering is currently viewed as everyone's responsibility yet no-one's responsibility.

Multidisciplinary sharing

The Faculty of Health Care and Social Work Studies is ideally placed to develop multidisciplinary shared teaching and learning. We are, however, constrained by 'semesterisation' within the University and the Regional requirement to produce a specified number of qualified nurses bi-annually. If we are to succeed in the development of 'fit for practice' multidisciplinary professionals, we must foster collaboration with our faculty colleagues to overcome these challenging but not insurmountable obstacles.

Teleconferencing

The University of Salford, in partnership with a commercial company and the City of Salford, has funded a multisite information technology project. Within this project is the opportunity for the Department of Nursing to develop teleconferencing facilities that will allow interaction between groups of students in the Skills Centre and students together with a lecturer and a patient in a clinical area within a local Trust. Computer hardware is available that, when utilising the immense cabling network now available to current and potential users, can create 'reality' and 'virtual reality', to the obvious advantage of those willing to explore the concepts. With the development of such projects, skills teaching can be enhanced, to the benefit of all concerned, especially our students, who long for patient contact but who must be taught safe practice.

Conclusion

The development of the skills workshops has been a valuable learning experience that has emphasised the value of negotiation, patience and quiet diplomacy. The positive effects of the workshops have been worth all the effort. Clinical managers report that their staff are aware of a distinct difference in the students in terms of their capabilities in the clinical area. Students are reporting that they feel confident when experiencing clinical practice for the first time. These views are different from those of previous students, who were much more apprehensive and felt ill prepared for their practice.

Creating reality for our students is a vital aspect of nurse education and one which we ignore at our peril.

References

Elkan, R and Robinson, J (1991) *The Implementation of Project 2000 in a District Health Authority; the Effect on the Nursing Service: An Interim Report.* Nottingham: Department of Nursing Studies, University of Nottingham.

Gomez, G E and Gomez, E A (1987) Learning of psychomotor skills: laboratory versus patient care setting. *Journal of Nursing Education* **26**(1): 20–4.

Jowett, S, Walton, I and Payne, S (1994) *Challenges and Changes in Nurse Education: A Study of the Implementation of Project 2000.* Slough: NFER.

O'Neill, A and McCall, J M (1996) Objectively assessing nursing practices: a curricular development. *Nurse Education Today* **16**: 121–6.

Neary, M (1994) Teaching practical skills in colleges. *Nursing Standard* **8**(27): 35–8.

Studdy, S, Nicol, M and Fox-Hiley, A (1994) Teaching and learning clinical skills. Part 1: Development of a multidisciplinary skills centre. *Nurse Education Today* **14**: 177–85.

United Kingdom Central Council for Nursing, Midwifery and Health Visting (1986) *Project 2000: A New Preparation for Practice.* London: UKCC.

4

Teaching, Learning and Assessment Strategies

Maggie Nicol and Carol Bavin

Introduction

As discussed in Chapter 1, the introduction of the Project 2000 Diploma programme meant that students spent much less time in the hospital ward setting, where they had traditionally learnt and practised their clinical skills. Clinical placements became more varied, and less time was spent in each, resulting in student complaints that they felt inadequate and unable to function as part of the team. Skills teaching had to become more structured and subsequent learning more focused in order to enable students to make the best use of their clinical placements. It is important to give students a baseline on which to build and enable them to recognise quality practice when they see it. This chapter describes how an interprofessional skills facility was developed to meet this need and outlines the way in which clinical skills teaching is addressed within the pre-registration programmes. Self-directed learning, through independent access to the Skills Centre, supported by 'in-house' instructional videos, is discussed, as is the use of the OSCE for the assessment of clinical competence.

The Skills Centre at St Bartholomew's

The Skills Centre at St Bartholomew's is an interprofessional initiative between the School of Nursing and Midwifery and the Medical School. The joint nature of this initiative has proved to be very important. Being the first of its kind in the UK, not only has it attracted a great deal of attention, but also, more importantly, funding. Funding has been provided almost exclusively by the Special Trustees of St Bartholomew's Hospital. They provided most of the building costs (£1.3 million) and the running costs for a period of 5 years (£1.25 million over 5 years). The Centre comprises: a simulated hospital ward; a simulated community setting; two multipurpose teaching laboratories; a range of models and simulators; a fully equipped communication skills suite; and video recording and playback facilities in both the clinical and communication skills areas (Dacre *et al.*, 1996).

There are four full-time members of staff at the Centre: a manager, a technician, a clinical skills teacher and a communication skills teacher. The two teaching posts are designed to develop teaching and self-directed learning within the Centre, and although they work with the academic staff of both Schools, they do not 'take over' teaching that would otherwise be provided by lecturers. They are primarily responsible for expanding the use of facilities within the Centre, producing self-directed learning materials, and for the development of interprofessional initiatives.

The Skills Centre is a new addition on the roof of an existing building belonging to the Medical School, but the new floor is seen as 'neutral' territory, an important consideration in interprofessional initiatives. It is housed in a building adjacent to St Bartholomew's Hospital, which is close to the main site of the School of Nursing and Midwifery (but not the other larger site) and was close to the Medical School. However, much change has occurred since it was built, and its future is now less certain owing to changes in clinical activity at St Bartholomew's Hospital, and the merger of the Medical School, with the result that it is now based several miles away.

In the initial stages, a steering group headed by the Deans of both Schools led the development. The chair alternated between the Schools and the steering group consisted of senior representatives (clinical and teaching) from each School as well as those involved in overseeing the building and so on. Within the School of Nursing, a lecturer in clinical skills was appointed (0.5 of the post funded by the Trustees and 0.5 by the School) to lead the initiative. This lecturer worked closely with a senior lecturer in the Medical School to plan and develop the Skills Centre and teaching opportunities within it. The lecturer in clinical skills also chairs a Caring Skills Group in the School of Nursing. This group comprises senior lecturers and lecturers representing Adult, Child and Mental Health branches, all of whom have close links with and regularly practise in the clinical areas. One remit of the group is to identify the skills to be included in the pre-registration programmes and the learning outcomes for each session. Members of this group are involved in most of the skills teaching.

Teaching and learning strategies

There are regular, planned clinical skills sessions throughout the pre-registration programme and in many post-registration programmes, particularly the short courses such as phlebotomy, taking cervical smears and suturing. A new undergraduate Diploma/Degree curriculum recognised the need for more time to be spent on clinical skills teaching, and an additional hour per week was allocated to the first 12-week module (Module A). In this module, students have 3 hours per week devoted to clinical skills: a 1-hour 'lead' lecture that covers the theory underpinning the skill(s) and a 2-hour small-group session that builds on the lead lecture but focuses very much on the practical aspects. The introduction of the lead lecture has meant that the practical sessions, which are designed to focus on one or two related clinical skills, can be devoted to demonstration and 'hands-on' practice by the students. Throughout the remainder of the CFP, students have varying amounts of clinical skills teaching according to the learning outcomes of each module.

During the branch programmes, it is mainly the Adult branch that uses the Centre. Because of the volume of teaching and the fact that the Skills Centre is shared with medical students, not all skills teaching can be accommodated within it. Two practical rooms (on other sites) and a 'manual handling' room are also used on a regular basis.

The Skills Centre is designed to provide a safe but realistic environment in which to learn and practise clinical skills. It is designed to simulate real clinical practice so that students learn skills in the context of real patient/client care and are better able to transfer them to the real care setting. Building on other parts of the course such as anatomy and physiology, pharmacology and nursing concepts and theories, skills are taught using the Integrated Skills Teaching Model (Nicol *et al.*, 1996), which is designed to encourage students to link theory and practice in the context of patient/client care. The development of nursing skills is planned throughout the 3-year programme and is detailed in the Schedule of Skills Development (Studdy *et al.*, 1994). This shows the skills required and the level of competence expected at various points in the programme.

The use of simulation is an important feature of the Skills Centre. All non-invasive skills are practised by students on each other, with the advantage that students learn not only how to perform the skill, but also how it feels to be a patient. It also encourages them to focus on normal physiology before progressing to potentially abnormal signs with real patients. Cohorts are divided into groups of 20–24 students, which with the large cohorts (200–250 students twice a year), means up to 11 small groups per week. This creates a considerable teacher demand, particularly as most sessions require two or even three teachers. Students are allocated to branch-specific groups at the beginning of the course. In order to ensure that the CFP is 'common' to all branches and does not become 'adult' focused, efforts are made to ensure that one of the lecturers teaching clinical skills to the Child and Mental Health groups has the appropriate professional background.

Caring Skills Workbook

The introduction of the lead lecture followed by small group practical sessions meant that students could be encouraged to contribute more towards their own learning and understanding of the various skills. The aim of the workbook is to encourage students to reflect on the lead lecture and seek out information or explore ideas in preparation for the small group sessions. It provides an overview of the skills addressed during the 12-week module and reminds the student that, although necessarily taught separately, the skills should not been seen in isolation but as part of the holistic process of nursing. It also stresses the relevance of other aspects of the course, such as biology, sociology, psychology and communication skills.

Each session is allocated two pages of the workbook, which allows space for the student to write the answers to a number of 'trigger' questions and make additional notes during small group teaching. The questions are designed to prompt the student to: seek out new information; recall previous knowledge or information provided in the lead lecture; relate physiology to themselves; or imagine how it might feel to be a patient. For example, for the session on respiratory observations, students are given the following trigger questions:

- What do the following terms mean: dyspnoea; peak flow; haemoptysis; bronchodilator; apnoea; Cheyne–Stokes respirations; expectoration?
- When completely out of breath (for example, after running fast), what position do people adopt to make breathing easier?
- List the structures involved in breathing, from nose to alveoli.

For the session on assisting with personal cleansing and dressing, the relevant questions are:

- Imagine that you are unable to get out of bed and have to be washed in bed by a nurse. How do you think you would feel? What would you like the nurse to consider?
- How should wash-bowls be cleaned and stored to prevent infection?
- Try holding your toothbrush in your non-dominant hand. How easy is it to clean your teeth?
- Is it possible to have your hair washed if you are confined to bed?

For the session on nutrition and feeding, the trigger questions are:

- It has been said that patients in hospital do not eat enough. Why do you think this might happen?
- Imagine that you are unable to move and have to be fed by a nurse. What would you like the nurse to consider?
- Think about your own eating habits and usual diet. Is it healthy? What is your Body Mass Index (BMI)? Is it within the recommended range?
- List the structures, from mouth to anus, involved in the digestion of food?

Students are advised to allow about an hour to complete the activities during their independent study, and are encouraged to use a range of resources, such as the library, computer packages and newspapers, as well as themselves and their friends. In the small group sessions, the lecturer uses the students' contributions as the basis for discussion and provides the 'correct' answers.

Evaluation of the workbook by students has been very positive. Most said that they had used it and found it useful particularly when revising for the Module A OSCE described later in this chapter. The generous space provided for notes meant that it could also be used during the sessions themselves.

Independent access by students

In order to encourage students to take responsibility for the development of their clinical skills, they are given opportunities for independent access to the Centre to further practise and maintain their skills. Students are required to book themselves into the Skills Centre and are provided with the relevant learning materials for the clinical skills they have chosen to practise. These include models and simulators (for example, injection buttocks) or equipment such as thermometers, sphygmomanometers or urine-testing equipment. A worksheet and/or instructional video that outlines the skill is also provided. The videos are 7–10 minutes long and have been produced in the Skills Centre by the technician and the authors. Students are encouraged to view the video in its entirety first in order to encourage them to appreciate the whole skill and the logical progression of the stages within it. The videos have proved very popular with the students because they can pause or replay parts as they practise the skill at their own speed until they feel confident. They are encouraged to book practice sessions in pairs or threes together so that they can help and support each other and also act as each other's patient where necessary.

The independent access is designed to be self-directed, so there is no teacher present. However, because students will be handling needles and other sharps, all Skills Centre staff have a knowledge of first aid in the event of an accident, and there is a Minor Injuries Centre within the same building. For security reasons, all materials, especially videos, are checked in and out by Centre staff, and students are required to provide their ID cards as security. Initially, students were reluctant to work on their own and wanted someone to teach them. However, as they became used to the idea and used the teaching materials, they soon found that they did not need a teacher. Independent access is designed to provide opportunities to practise the skill and to develop confidence and dexterity, as a supplement to the teaching programme rather than to replace it.

Manual handling and moving skills are addressed in a lead lecture (1 hour) followed by three practical sessions (2 hours each) in Module A which require high levels of supervision (3 lecturers for 20–24 students) to ensure safety. Students are not permitted to practise manual handling and moving skills during independent access as it is not considered safe do this without teacher supervision. To provide supervision would mean that teaching hours would have to be identified, and this is currently not possible. However, the importance of safe manual handling and the students' need for practice is recognised, not least by the students themselves. Two stations testing manual handling and moving skills are currently included in the Module A OSCE described below. This is a formative OSCE, so, where necessary, the lecturer provides guidance to ensure safe prac-tice. The need to provide the facilities to allow students to practise these vital skills safely before they come into contact with patients and clients is recognised, but the School has yet to find a solution to this problem.

Video production

The instructional videos have been produced in the Skills Centre using two overhead cameras with tilt and zoom facilities, and one free-standing camcorder. The camcorder is used to record the wide shot and sound throughout, and the other cameras provide close-up shots. The presenters are experienced nurse lecturers who regularly teach clinical skills. This enables the videos to be spontaneous and unscripted, resulting in a more natural presentation. Each video is 7–10 minutes long, and making them involves the lecturers for an average of three half-day sessions in the Skills Centre. The first session involves rehearsing the skill in order to determine the position of the cameras and to identify the close-up shots. This session also enables the technician to become acquainted with the skill, and the lecturers to clarify details and points that need to be emphasised. The draft video is then edited by the technician, to be reviewed at the beginning of the second session. Changes to camera angles, close-ups, 'script', continuity and so on are decided and set up ready for the final recording. Two or three takes are usually necessary before the presenters are wholly satisfied. In the third session, the edited video is reviewed and final adjustments are made. The technician then creates a short pictorial title page and adds viewing information, credits and so on.

The resulting video provides students with the opportunity to have access to a teacher demonstration in their own time as often as they wish. When used in teaching sessions, the video can be shown to 'set the scene' and also provide students with close-up views that are often not possible in a demonstration. In addition to supporting self-directed learning, the videos have also proved useful for lecturers who wish to update their own practice.

Assessment of clinical skills

The assessment of clinical skills throughout the programme is mostly through Practice-based Assessments (learning outcomes) within the students' clinical placements, which, except for the first placement, are summative. In addition to the Practice-based Assessments, students have three OSCEs (Harden and Gleeson, 1979) during the 3-year programme. The first is at the end of the first module (Module A), which is prior to their first clinical placement, the second is in Module B immediately after the first clinical placement, and the third comes during the Branch programme.

Module A OSCE

At this stage (3 months into the CFP), students have had no clinical experience but have been taught a range of fundamental nursing skills within the Skills Centre. The OSCE is formative and is designed to introduce students to this form of assessment, and to test their ability to perform these skills safely prior to contact with real patients. As is traditional, the OSCE is arranged so that students rotate through a number of stations at timed intervals. To accommodate the large number of students, they are in pairs, which means that they can act as each other's patient where necessary.

Using the Levels of Skills Acquisition devised within the School (Nicol *et al.*, 1996), students are required to demonstrate Foundation Level performance (Box 4.1) in a number of skills that they will be able to develop further in their clinical placements. These include: temperature, pulse and blood pressure recording; urine testing; emptying a catheter bag; peak flow measurement; hand-washing; assisting a patient to use a commode; basic life support; and the principles of manual handling and moving. The OSCE has 12 stations so that 12 pairs of students can undertake the OSCE at the same time. Students are allowed 8 minutes (4 minutes each) at each station, so 24 students can thus be accommodated within a 2-hour timetabled session. Of the 12 stations, 5 are assessed by lecturers, 2 are designed so that the students assess each other, thus

BOX 4.1

LEVELS OF CLINICAL SKILLS DEVELOPMENT

A: Foundation
- The student is able to demonstrate psychomotor components of the skill
- Performance is slow and lacks co-ordination
- The student is able to identify the cognitive and affective components of the skill

B: Safe and accurate performance in the Skills Centre
- The student is able to demonstrate accuracy in the skill but not necessarily speed
- Psychomotor dexterity is demonstrated
- Awareness of the cognitive and affective components of the skill is demonstrated

C: Safe and accurate performance under direct supervision
- The student is able to demonstrate accuracy in the skill but not necessarily speed
- Psychomotor dexterity is demonstrated
- Awareness of the cognitive and affective components of the skill is demonstrated

D: Safe and accurate performance with indirect supervision
- Performance of the skill is accurate, co-ordinated, effective and affective
- The student is able to adapt in response to changes in the care situation
- Cognitive and affective components of the skill are integrated
- The student is aware of his or her limitations and seeks help and advice as appropriate
- Performance at this level is 'competent'

E: Skill mastery
- Psychomotor aspects of the skill no longer require conscious thought
- Cognitive and affective components are highly developed
- Performance experience is confident, efficient and responsive to situational cues
- Reflection is central to practice at this level

(Nicol *et al.*, 1996)

developing skills of peer assessment, and 4 are quiz-type stations. These cover areas such as nutrition, manual handling, the identification of equipment and the definition of terms such as haematuria, and students may discuss their answers with each other. There is also one rest station that provides an opportunity for refreshment, a visit to the toilet and so on. At the end of the OSCE, students complete a self-evaluation form that is designed to encourage them to reflect on their level of ability and identify learning needs.

The OSCE is followed by a feedback session for the whole cohort at the end of the week, in which students receive their OSCE checklists with written comments on the teacher-assessed stations, and the answers to the quiz questions.

Overall evaluation of the OSCE by lecturers and students has been positive. Students, although nervous, generally perform to the required standard. As expected, they lack speed and dexterity in the various skills, but most are able to demonstrate an understanding of how to perform the skill. As the OSCE occurs prior to their first clinical placement, this allows them to identify areas in which they need more practice and support from their clinical assessor. The OSCE also encourages students to take clinical skills seriously. Attendance at the OSCE is excellent, and large numbers of students use the independent access facility to practise skills beforehand. The OSCE remains teacher intensive, but by including stations that do not require a teacher, the demand is reduced. This also means more variety and less stress for the students as they are not being observed at every station. The OSCE not only provides valuable feedback for students on how their skills are developing, but also guidance for lecturers regarding the clinical skills content of the programme.

Module B OSCE

This takes place immediately after the first clinical placement, which comprises 4 weeks (20 days) continuous placement in an adult hospital ward. This OSCE is designed to test the way in which students' skills are developing, but unlike the Module A OSCE, it is also designed to test the integration of clinical and communication skills and the demonstration of concepts such as respect and maintaining privacy and dignity. This is a summative OSCE, so students are on their own rather than in pairs, and perform the required skills on a simulated patient. Also, in order to demonstrate the integration of clinical and communication skills, students do not move through a number of stations but remain at one station caring for one patient. The lecturer wears a uniform and acts as if working with the student on the ward. This is felt to provide a realistic representation of the clinical situation.

The stations are designed so that each student is required to demonstrate a safe level of practice (Level B/C, see Box 4.1) in the fundamental skills of temperature, pulse and blood pressure recording. Each student is also required to perform one or two other skills, which vary from station to station. These include urinalysis, emptying a catheter bag and assisting with mobility or elimination needs. This approach differs from the Module A OSCE in which all students are required to perform all the skills. However, students do not know their allocated station prior to the OSCE, so do not know in advance which particular skills they will be asked to perform. This is consistent with other forms of assessment in which only a sample of the curriculum rather than all the content is tested. To pass the OSCE, students are expected to perform at Level C – *safe and accurate performance under direct supervision*.

It is stressed that students should know when to seek help and ask the lecturer to assist or check an observation in the same way as they would ask a qualified nurse on clinical placement. A student who is unable to hear the blood pressure, for example, but has demonstrated a knowledge of the technique and has asked the lecturer to check the reading, would be considered safe and thus achieve a pass. Failure to recognise when he or she has done something incorrectly, or failure to record the correct reading without asking for this to be checked, will result in a fail. This enables students to make mistakes as a result of inexperience or nerves but to redeem themselves by recognising that they have made a mistake or that they need assistance.

Because this is a summative OSCE, students are video recorded at the station. It is not possible to achieve quality recordings, particularly of sound, at all the stations during the OSCE. However, it is possible to achieve this for second attempts because, as there are a smaller number of students, the stations can be arranged in such a way that quality visual and audio recording is possible. Students are initially concerned about being recorded, but because the cameras are ceiling mounted and very unobtrusive, students quickly forget about them, and it has not been found to affect their performance. The recording of the re-sit enables the OSCE to be moderated, and the tapes may also be sent to an external examiner, particularly in the event of failure leading to discontinuation from the course. It will also enable students to see where they have gone wrong and make the OSCE more objective. A sample of stations at the first attempt are 'moderated' by a senior lecturer to ensure consistency between lecturers and throughout the day.

Branch programme OSCE

An OSCE is currently being developed to assess students in their third year and will include the need to plan and prioritise care as well as to demonstrate competence in a range of skills. It is planned that the OSCE will be linked to an examination involving a reflective essay in which students are required to demonstrate a knowledge and understanding of the theory and principles underpinning the care they have given.

Interprofessional education

Opportunities for shared learning between nurses and medical students are being explored. A small but very successful interprofessional study day has been run several times (see Freeth and Nicol, 1998, for a detailed description). This brings a small group of newly qualified staff nurses and fifth-year medical students together and is led by the senior lecturer for clinical skills and a consultant physician. Using a realistic patient scenario as the focus, the participants teach each other clinical skills and discuss the care and management of the patient. All those involved enjoy the day and find it a valuable learning experience. It is now hoped that it can be developed and used by other lecturers and clinicians in order to reach larger numbers of participants.

The Skills Centre provides an ideal setting for the development of such initiatives, but it is recognised that, for interprofessional education to achieve its ultimate aim of improving teamwork and thus the quality of patient care, it is necessary for it to be continued in the real clinical setting. One such initiative that is currently being implemented is the development of an interprofessional training ward. This is a hospital ward specialising in rheumatology and orthopaedics, where senior students from nursing, medicine, physiotherapy and occupational therapy will work together under supervision and run the ward on a 24-hour basis. They will have interprofessional teaching sessions and reflective tutorials to explore professional relationships and how these influence patient care.

Conclusion

The Skills Centre has proved to be a successful initiative that has enabled us to deliver quality clinical skills teaching in a realistic but safe environment. The provision of independent access encourages and enables students to take responsibility for their own learning in the same way as they are expected to in other aspects of the course. It also allows them to practise and develop skills at their own speed, safe in the knowledge that mistakes do not matter. The Skills Centre provides an attractive, realistic simulation of practice that enables junior nurses to develop a wide range of fundamental nursing skills before exposure to real patients and clients. This means that students on placement feel part of the clinical team and have the confidence to make the best use of the valuable learning opportunities that are only found in the real clinical care setting.

The Skills Centre also has an important role to play in the development of advanced skills such as catheterisation and suturing, through the use of sophisticated models and simulators. Use of the Skills Centre by advanced practitioners is increasing, and simulated patients with a variety of pathologies are being recruited to enable them to develop, and be tested on, the skills of physical assessment.

Plans for the future include making further use of the video equipment for the self- and peer-assessment of learning. Both the clinical and the communications skills facilities are fully equipped with video recording equipment, but this has yet to be fully utilised, although it has been vital to the development of the instructional videos. The use of video playback by students as they develop their skills is something that is being explored. In certain skills, such as blood pressure recording or aseptic dressing technique, the video camera should provide valuable feedback to the student about his or her performance. It would also provide a valuable record of skills development over time. When students are worrying about how much they have to learn, it would be encouraging to be able to remind them just how much they have already achieved.

Evaluation of the Skills Centre is also vital. Part of the funding provides for a full-time senior lecturer in research in both the Nursing and Medical Schools. Research thus far has focused on the interprofessional nature of the initiative, but there is a real need to evaluate the impact of the Skills Centre on nursing education. All those who teach within it would argue that it is valuable, and verbal feedback from students suggests that it makes an important contribution to the development of skilled nurses. However, hard evidence in terms of positive outcomes for students, and eventually patients, may be needed to justify the expense.

References

Dacre, J, Nicol, M, Holroyd, D and Ingram, D (1996) The development of a clinical skills centre, *Journal of the Royal College of Physicians* **30**(4): 318–24.

Freeth, D and Nicol, M (1998) Learning clinical skills: an interprofessional approach. *Nurse Education Today* **18**: 455–61.

Harden, R and Gleeson, F (1979) Assessment of clinical competence using an objective structured clinical examination (OSCE), *Medical Education* **13**: 41–51.

Nicol, M, Fox-Hiley, A, Bavin, C and Sheng, R (1996) Assessment of clinical and communication skills: operationalizing Benner's model. *Nurse Education Today* **16**: 175–9.

Studdy, S, Nicol, M and Fox-Hiley, A (1994) Teaching and learning clinical skills. Part 1: Development of a multidisciplinary skills centre. Part 2: Development of a teaching model and schedule of skills development. *Nurse Education Today* **14**: 177–93.

5

A Healthcare Network Approach

Sally Glen and Iain McA Ledingham

Introduction

Towards the end of 1996, an opportunity presented itself to the University of Dundee to lay the foundation of an exciting, far-sighted and educationally sound collaborative education programme in healthcare practice, which included the establishment of a Healthcare Learning Network. This concept is based on the premise that knowledge development and acquisition are no longer bound by place and time but occur at any time and from any place (Figure 5.1).

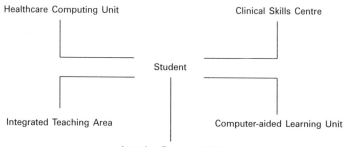

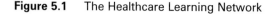

Figure 5.1   The Healthcare Learning Network

These shifts are enabled, to a large extent, by learning technologies that promote access and connectivity through voice, video and data lines. The Healthcare Learning Network facilitates access and connectivity to resources well beyond the traditional physical spaces of a 'learning lab' (Billings, 1996). The Healthcare Learning Network is a Faculty of Medicine, Dentistry and Nursing, Trust and community initiative. It allows medical, dental, nursing and midwifery students to acquire or refine a range of clinical and communication skills (Box 5.1).

BOX 5.1

CORE CLINICAL AND COMMUNICATION SKILLS

- Communication and history-taking skills
- Professional attitudes and awareness of the ethical basis of health and social care
- Assessment, physical examination and procedural skills
- Ethical awareness
- Essential care skills
- Resuscitation skills
- Critical thinking, reasoning and problem-solving skills
- Teamworking, organisation and management skills
- Information technology skills

Local determinants

The context of healthcare policy and the nature of healthcare itself has exerted a major influence on educational innovation and developments in relation to the teaching and learning of skills. As discussed in Chapter 1, shorter admissions to hospital, increased care in the community and reduced resources, fewer in-patients and a shorter length of stay have caused problems for the traditional apprenticeship system. In addition, teaching methods now place an increased emphasis on small group work and self-directed learning. There were also, simultaneously, important local determinants.

First, the Medical School implemented a new undergraduate curriculum during the academic year 1995–96. Preparation for the new curriculum involved the creation of a number of innovative physical resources. These included the Clinical Skills Centre, the Learning Resources Area, the Medical Disciplines Integration Area and the Computer Suite. Second, at the end of 1995, the Scottish Office offered the University of Dundee a contract for pre-registration nursing and midwifery education on the proviso that the curriculum contained substantial elements of multiprofessional education. Third, in September 1996, the School of Nursing and Midwifery was formed as a new School within a Faculty of Medicine, Dentistry and Nursing. One of the principal objectives of this landmark move was the development of multiprofessional education.

Clinical skills teaching, learning and research are seen as priority areas within the School of Nursing and Midwifery. Clinical skills teaching and learning also offer many opportunities for multiprofessional education and research within the context of a Healthcare Learning Network.

The Healthcare Learning Network

The Healthcare Learning Network is part of a collaboration between the University, local Trusts and the community. The principal aims are to:

- optimise the provision and facilitate the effective utilisation of educational resources
- promote the development of multiprofessional education and research relevant to healthcare practice.

In a variety of different settings, the Network encourages students, as they progress through their curricula, to acquire higher-level skills, for example collating, integrating, synthesising, analysing and evaluating data, using both traditional facilities and state-of-the-art computer-aided learning. These skills form the basis for the development of increasingly sophisticated problem-solving and decision-making abilities in a wide range of health and social care experiences. By means of internal links (with, for example, the Life-long Learning Centre, the Centre for Medical Education, the Surgical Skills Unit, and Tayside Centre for Primary Healthcare) and external links (with, for example, the Royal Colleges and other post-graduate bodies), the Network aims to ensure a clear continuity between undergraduate/pre-registration, post-graduate/post-registration and continuing healthcare education.

Clinical skills facility

The Clinical Skills Centre, called the Joint Learning Centre for Healthcare Practice, is strategically sited within the Dundee Teaching Hospitals Trust and is a purpose-built facility where students, lecturers and patients can work together in comfortable surroundings and realistic settings with appropriate privacy. In this way, students from all healthcare professions learn how to bridge the gap between theory and practice.

The Centre comprises two distinct but adjacent areas. One area consists of a ring of demonstration and communication rooms with, at its core, a small seminar suite, a smart bistro-style social space where information can be exchanged in an informal atmosphere, and a reception area. The layout of the individual rooms can be changed according to requirement. The other adjacent area consists of simulated client settings, for example home, child and adult/critical care. This area is also a fully equipped nursing and midwifery skills area. The latter has been designed to simulate up-to-date clinical hospital and community situations, and is equipped with the appropriate equipment and technology used in local NHS Trusts. This provision allows for nursing and midwifery nursing students to develop their confidence in handling equipment and to carry out nursing and midwifery skills prior to allocation to the placement areas. The focus of these two areas is to develop competencies in students prior to their experience in the practice placement areas.

Learning opportunities

A small multidisciplinary team, in collaboration with programme/route/module leaders, develops and co-ordinates the delivery of the learning programmes. A range of learning resources is utilised (Box 5.2).

BOX 5.2

LEARNING RESOURCES

- Anatomical models and monitors
- Diagnostic and therapeutic equipment
- Resuscitation equipment
- Computers and videos
- Telemedia links within and beyond the campus
- Simulated and real patients
- A simulated 'home setting', childcare setting and adult/critical care setting

---

Lecturers and lecturer-practitioners have a clear need to be up to date with current clinical practice as well as having a knowledge of the latest research pertaining to the skills being addressed. The lecturers are therefore all experienced professionals in active clinical practice. Common attributes include a general and integrative educational approach, and enthusiasm for and competence in small group teaching. Clinical competence and clinical credibility are clear key issues. Some might argue that this is nothing more than a return to the old-style 'practical room'. However, there are a number of fundamental differences. A holistic approach is emphasised using role play, and students can discuss decisions and priorities of care with the facilitator and their peers. Students are also encouraged to keep a record of their achievements in their Portfolio. This aids their clinical supervisors, mentors and preceptors to determine their learning needs.

Users of the Clinical Skills Centre include dental, medical, nursing and midwifery students at undergraduate and postgraduate levels. The Faculty of Medicine, Dentistry and Nursing places a high priority on the development of multiprofessional education and training, advancing a number of advantages in support of this approach:

- a richer educational environment for both students and teachers
- the development of mutual respect for, and understanding of, other professional groups
- a greater understanding among students of their own professional roles
- the efficient use of shared resources
- a better preparedness for post-registration work in multiprofessional teams
- the promotion of multiprofessional research activities.

Aims of the Healthcare Learning Network

The Faculty of Medicine, Dentistry and Nursing has articulated a number of aims related to the development of multiprofessional education (Box 5.3).

To address the aims outlined in Box 5.3, a programme of multiprofessional education and training among medical, dental, nursing and midwifery students was developed. It is based on the following principles:

- to use learning materials on a shared basis in courses with common foundations
- to explore the complementary and interdependent roles of the different professions
- to receive instruction, in a shared environment, on clinical skills performed in a collaborative manner
- to gain an experience of clinical problem-solving in a multiprofessional environment
- to have extended opportunities for multiprofessional learning in the post-qualification phase of education and training
- to facilitate integration between pre- and post-registration education.

BOX 5.3

UNIVERSITY OF DUNDEE FACULTY OF MEDICINE, DENTISTRY AND NURSING – AIMS OF MULTIPROFESSIONAL EDUCATION

1. To prepare students for multiprofessional working after qualification by:

   - improving the understanding of the roles of different health professionals
   - developing a respect for and communication with other professional groups
   - improving awareness of how professionals work in multi-disciplinary teams
   - developing shared attitudes towards patients/clients

2. To create a stimulating educational environment within the faculty by:

   - developing shared elements of teaching and learning
   - providing different perspectives of healthcare delivery and professional roles
   - sharing the experience of simulated clinical scenarios

3. To develop cost-effective educational strategies by:

   - the shared use of learning materials, library, staff resources, teaching premises and recreational facilities
   - innovative technology in the delivery and management of teaching and learning

---

Computer-assisted learning

Computer technology lends itself to a complementary role within the Skills Centre. Computer-assisted-learning (CAL) adds to the continual assessment and refinement of the teaching method because of a computer's ability to store users' responses and hence allow the identification of learning needs and individual user problems. Drug calculation programmes, for example, can reinforce present knowledge and rectify mistakes. Anatomical and physiological programmes can present the student with realistic and detailed three-dimensional images of the human body and thus assist them in being able to understand the pathophysiological process. All students have access to e-mail within the School and are therefore able to submit work to, and receive feedback from, academic staff. Lecturers are also encouraged to utilise CAL packages within their mainstream teaching as opposed to seeing CAL packages as purely a revision tool or a student-directed resource.

This strategy requires appropriate staff development sessions to assist lecturers to expand the use of information technology (IT) within the classroom and to explore ways of doing so. There has of course been a dramatic increase in the availability of CD-Rom-based materials over the past few years. Much of this material comes in the form of databases that allow students to access information and/or materials to support their learning. CD-Roms are widely used by students, and this practice is encouraged. The School is also working towards ensuring that all problem-based learning packages are networked and permit student self-directed learning during and outside class time. This has resource implications related to the need for computer terminals within classrooms and the appropriate software.

The School is working towards integrating IT with distance and open learning. The main goal of this project is the development of an ISDN network of linked multimedia computers that enable students to access internet-based learning materials from locations distant from the School. Video conferencing is an integral part of the project to ensure that lecturer support is provided for students (Pope, 1995; Billings, 1996; McKenzie, 1996). However, CAL will never replace the role of the educator. It is important to recognise that only human perception can understand a student's personality, strengths and weaknesses. Computers can enhance the effectiveness of teaching methods, but they cannot replace them.

Assessment of students

The assessment of student performance is achieved by a number of methods, most being variants of the OSCE (as described in Chapter 4). A series of realistic 'stations' tests student competencies in a broad range of challenging, task-based situations. Feedback to students is an integral part of the learning process.

Simulated patients

'Simulated patients' are dedicated volunteers from all walks of life, of all ages and with all levels of fitness and health. All simulated patients are recruited by advertising in the local newspaper. The future challenge for the Faculty is not in recruiting simulated patients but in retaining them. Simulated patients undergo a variety of specific training programmes and in turn help us to train students. The use of simulated rather than real patients offers the following advantages; it:

- controls the complexity of the learning situation
- allows mistakes to be made within a safe environment
- encourages direct feedback
- is independent of 'real' patient availability
- directly involves members of the local community in the healthcare learning process.

Evaluation of the Network

Evaluation, which is ongoing throughout the Healthcare Learning Network development, has been largely qualitative and directed towards obtaining the subjective opinions of students and teachers. Evaluation is essential in order to identify which subject/tasks are better learned multiprofessionally and which are better learned apart. Indeed, the uniprofessional learning of technical skills is probably as efficient as the multiprofessional; thus beneficial outcomes are more likely to be in the area of attitude change. There is a need for further research in relation to whether exposure to this teaching approach increases conceptual and analytic ability, and clinical judgement. More importantly, in the longer term, it is important to determine whether students exposed to this method of teaching are 'fit for purpose' and able to deliver and improve the quality of care. There are of course difficulties associated with evaluating successful outcomes, particularly in relation to the long-term outcome of improved patient care. Such evidence may prove crucial in the current political and economic climate because Clinical Skills Centres are an expensive alternative.

Future developments

The School and the Faculty have recently implemented Problem-based Learning (PBL) as a learning strategy to facilitate the learning of clinical skills. It encourages a cognitive style in students, such as analytical thinking, that is conducive to higher education. These are the skills that enable students to make sense of the world in which they operate. The process of teaching skills using a PBL approach has proved to be a significant challenge for lecturers, some of whom find this approach quite demanding; others will consider it to be part of their current repertoire and find it much easier to adapt (Murray, 1997). The use of PBL is in the early stages of development, so it is too early to make definitive statements relating to its success. However, initial evaluation by students and staff is very positive.

Conclusion

The Healthcare Learning Network complements 'real' clinical experience, exposure to which occurs concurrently in conventional practice settings. Students can develop their affective, psychomotor and cognitive skills in a less threatening environment, and lecturers are able to relate theory to practice more successfully. Students are also constantly reminded that knowledge is not static and that their practice must, therefore, evolve in the light of research-based evidence. The Healthcare Learning Network appears to offer enormous potential, not only in terms of enhancing current nurse and midwifery education programmes, but also in promoting multiprofessional teaching and learning. The exploration and adoption of such strategies nationally may, in the longer term, serve to enhance collaborative working.

References

Billings, D M (1996) Learning centres. *Computers in Nursing* **14**(2): 80–7.

McKenzie, B C (1996) *Medicine and the Internet*. Oxford: Oxford University Press.

Murray, I D (1997) Problem-based learning and the integration of a nursing curriculum. In Conway, J, Fisher, R, Sherridan-Burns, L and Ryan, G (eds) *Research and Development in PBL*, Vol. 4: *Integrity, Innovation and Integration*. Australian PBL Network: Sydney, Australia.

Pope, I (1995) *Internet UK*. London: Prentice-Hall.

6

A Portfolio Approach

Isabelle Whaite, Rose Allen and Dorothy Jones

Introduction

This chapter outlines an approach to the teaching and learning of clinical skills that forms an integral part of the overall clinical assessment strategy adopted in the BSc (Hons) Nursing pre-registration curriculum. Key values that have influenced the design and development of the clinical assessment strategy and tools are discussed, together with development work currently being undertaken in translating these into action. The search for a suitable model and strategy for teaching, learning and assessing nursing students in practice is briefly discussed, as is an outline of the model which is currently being tested. A key tool designed for formative assessment is the Portfolio, which includes a section for clinical skills learning. By adopting this approach, it is hoped that a balance between students 'learning' and 'doing' in practice can be achieved.

Key values

Central key values stated in the BSc (Hons) Nursing pre-registration curriculum document were of major significance in formulating the clinical assessment strategy and in influencing the design and development of tools for learning and assessment in clinical practice. They are reflected in the value statements extracted from the curriculum (Box 6.1).

BOX 6.1

VALUE STATEMENTS EXTRACTED FROM THE CURRICULUM

- Nursing theory and practice are equally valued
- Learning about nursing and learning how to learn are equally important
- Practice is central to nurse education rather than peripheral to it
- Nursing competence is more than the ability to carry out technical skills and tasks in practice
- Lecturers in nursing, clinical practitioners and students have equal responsibility for teaching and learning in practice

The equal value placed on theory and practice is demonstrated in the curriculum modules that are designed to integrate the two. Clinical learning outcomes are written for each module, and are designed to assess both theory and practice.

The theory–practice gap perceived by some nursing students, teachers and clinical practitioners (Allen, 1992; Butterworth, 1994; Wilson-Thomas, 1995) would seem to indicate a tendency towards the compartmentalisation of knowledge by students, knowledge acquired through study and knowledge acquired through experience being contained within two separate compartments (Argyris and Schön, 1974). Although this compartmentalisation may be understandable early in a programme, a key question is whether students are enabled, through current approaches to teaching, learning and assessment, to begin to reduce this gap as they progress through the programme. A knowledge-based curriculum that does not enable students to use their knowledge to inform and enhance learning in practice would have serious shortcomings.

The belief in the centrality of practice in nurse education is demonstrated through the development of a clinical link role for Faculty-based lecturers. This is seen as an essential strategy to ground nurse education more firmly in practice (RCN, 1993; ENB, 1995). The focus of the role is primarily to prepare and provide continued support for qualified clinical staff in undertaking their teaching and assessing roles in clinical practice. Lecturers in nursing have joint responsibility with clinical assessors and students for teaching and learning in practice. Clinical assessors and their teams are the key people in establishing and maintaining a learning environment that will facilitate students' learning in practice. Several studies have identified indicators that positively influence learning in clinical environments (Fretwell, 1980; Ogier, 1982; Orton, 1981, 1993). More recent studies would seem to indicate that students do not always experience an environment conducive to learning. Factors such as lack of support, not feeling safe, not being recognised for themselves as persons and judgmental attitudes are some of the reasons given by students as contributing to an environment not conducive to learning (Ace Project, 1992; Phillips *et al.*, 1994; May *et al.*, 1997).

As the previous three chapters illustrate, many Schools of Nursing have re-introduced the concept of the practical room to ensure that clinical skills teaching is valued and students are able to practise the skills they need in a safe environment. However, this approach requires a large amount of human and financial resources, especially with large cohorts of students. Rather than following this trend, our Faculty decided to address the problems encountered by students in clinical practice by improving the structure and opportunities for learning in the practice areas through the development of the Portfolio.

Competence

In the BSc (Hons) Nursing curriculum, competence is defined as 'the knowledge, skills, attitudes, energy, experience, motivation and ability to integrate theory with practice resulting in effective action to be achieved in a constantly changing, intricate and complex context'. It is also 'a continuous process of striving to improve the effectiveness of professional action and acquiring the disposition of valuing this process and the skills of learning how to learn'. Thus, in addition to skills and techniques, it refers to the student's developing ability to integrate knowledge that informs and enhances learning in practice. This also needs to be measured in clinical practice assessment.

While the acquisition of clinical skills is a highly valued element of professional competence, it is recognised that competence in nursing also includes all of the elements discussed above. The overall strategy adopted in the programme for the teaching, learning and assessment of competence provides a framework to guide student learning in the acquisition of all of these elements, including learning how to learn and the acquisition of clinical skills. The dangers of clinical staff using criteria that define competence too narrowly, limiting it to technical skills and tasks, are reported (Phillips *et al.*, 1994; May *et al.*, 1997).

Clinical assessment

In the search for a suitable model and strategy that would embrace the key values, an extensive literature review was undertaken of clinical assessment strategies, models and instruments currently in use within nursing programmes in the United Kingdom. Although many clinical assessment tools have been developed and reported in the literature, few appear to have been evaluated, and their effectiveness is thus unclear (Coates and Chambers, 1992; Phillips *et al.*, 1994; May *et al.*, 1997). In the absence of any 'tried and tested' tool being available, it was decided to design and test a clinical assessment instrument through an action research approach within the BSc (Hons) Nursing pre-registration programme. The theoretical framework adopted for the development of the instrument is based on the findings of a study undertaken to explore the nature of medical expertise and the stages of progression from novice to expert status (Patel and Groen, 1991). The effectiveness of the clinical assessment instrument is being measured in five key areas: its value in practice in being able to distinguish between the various levels of progressing practice competence at each key progress stage in the programme; its adaptability for use in a variety of settings; its applicability to a variety of clinical settings of varying durations; whether it makes clinical assessment more objective; and whether it facilitates continuous learning and assessment. The instrument will clearly need to be tested and modified repeatedly before one can achieve a more reliable way of assessing competence that includes all of the elements already discussed, particularly the integration of knowledge with ability, learning to learn and the acquisition of clinical skills.

Two key tools have been designed: the Module Assessment Record and the Portfolio. The Module Assessment Record is designed for use at the summative stage when the assessor makes a judgement about the student's achievement against the relevant module learning outcomes. The Portfolio is designed to guide students and provide support and formative assessment. It is through the formative assessment process that clinical skills learning is promoted, structured and profiled throughout the entire programme. Included within the student's nursing practice Portfolio is the clinical skills schedule, through which the student is required to build a profile of clinical skills development and achievement as he or she progresses through the course programme. Formative and summative assessments are equally important elements within the overall clinical assessment instrument; however, for the purpose of this chapter, further discussion will focus on the design and development of the Portfolio with particular reference to the Clinical Skills Schedule.

The Portfolio

The Portfolio is intended as a tool and framework to facilitate the formative process of learning and the assessment of progressing practice competence. It is divided into nine sections: Learning Contracts; Progress Records; Module Learning Outcomes; Evidence Collection; Schedule of Clinical Skills; Modular Reflection; Self-assessment and Review of Learning; Transferable Skills and Learning Statements; and Record of Practice Experience. It will also provide the student with a record of achievement. It is intended as a vehicle to create opportunities for discussion between students, lecturers and clinical practitioners, and to engender supportive partnerships through which learning and the development of practice can take place. This could provide a rich repository of learning for all.

Unlike traditional pre-Project 2000 curricula, in which students were often seen as 'pairs of hands' in the clinical areas, practice areas are selected on the basis that they will provide students with access to the necessary experience required to achieve module learning outcomes. Module learning outcomes provide students, lecturers and assessors with the focus for learning, which is then translated into the learning contracts. The process approach to the assessment of practice requires Portfolio development, goal identification and action-planning on the student's part. Central to this process is the Learning Contract (Figure 6.1), which the student begins to prepare prior to each practice placement in readiness to be negotiated with the clinical assessor at the commencement of the placement. Students are expected to work in partnership with the module lecturers and clinical assessors in the process of reviewing learning and progress in relation to the clinical learning outcomes. The process is designed to identify strengths, learning needs and skills requiring further development in practice, and how to apply previous knowledge in new areas of practice.

The Learning Contract

The review of learning and the diagnosis of learning needs play a crucial role in the contract-setting negotiations. The Learning Contract is an agreed written document that states identified learning needs in relation to the module's clinical learning outcomes. It also includes a plan that specifies strategy, targets and methods to be used in order to achieve learning, together with the resources needed. At the beginning of the course, students need a substantial amount of help and support from module lecturers and clinical assessors in preparing and negotiating a learning contract. Module lecturers are responsible for facilitating the students' achievement of both theoretical and clinical module learning outcomes. This approach is central to the overall teaching and learning strategy adopted in the curriculum. The focus for teaching is facilitating students' integration of learning through academic study with learning in and from practice experience. The key tool for guiding and supporting learning in practice is the Portfolio.

LEARNING CONTRACT   **MODULE** . . . .

                    YEAR . . . .

Name of Student . . . .

Name of Assessor(s) . . . . Ward/Unit . . . .

                    . . . . Ward/Unit . . . .

Identified learning needs including skills

see: Skills Schedule
Module Clinical Outcomes and Transferable Skills
Module Reflection and Review of Learning
Review of Progress Record

Action plan – Include objectives, resources needed and the nature of
evidence to be collected

Dates for ongoing assessment of learning
(at least two formative meetings in each placement)

Date of Contract . . . . End of Contract Date . . . .

Signature of Student . . . .

Signature of Assessor . . . .

Figure 6.1   The Learning Contract

LEVEL 1

Module title: Philosophy and Ethics for Nursing

- Identify and use different approaches and tools to assist the development of reflective practice
- Explore and describe the nature and pattern of current nursing knowledge through reading, observation, conversation and debate with colleagues
- Examine and describe examples of different frameworks for care and their underpinning values and beliefs
- Describe the concept of professionalism in order to understand the changing contexts, conflicts and dilemmas that nurses experience in day-to-day practice
- Identify and consider national and international legal frameworks within which nursing and healthcare services operate
- Explore and describe the nature of power and control in relation to nursing as a profession and day-to-day nursing practice
- Explore moral theory, principles and tools supporting ethical decision-making in practice
- Consider and reflect upon caring as a base and framework for legal, professional and ethical practice and decision-making

Clinical Learning Outcomes

- Identify in practice, through conversation, observation and debate, the varied sources of knowledge used in everyday clinical practice
- Explore, describe and discuss one model of care identified in practice
- Identify an ethical conflict/dilemma from the placement setting and describe the underlying issues that have created the dilemma and that influence potential resolution
- Consider the ideal of 'duty of care' in practice and identify nursing activities that support the concept in practice

Core Transferable Skills

- *Problem-solving:* Consider what factors create ethical and moral dilemmas
- *Communications and interpersonal skills:* Explore the use of touch in practice and identify values that support or prevent its use
- *Management of self:* Clarify personal values that support a personal philosophy of care

---

Figure 6.2 Module learning outcomes

The student is required to work with module lecturers and clinical assessors to determine the nature, level and range of written evidence to be produced by the student while on practice placement to demonstrate the achievement of module learning outcomes. An example of the clinical skills associated with the Philosophy and Ethics for Nursing module is shown in Box 6.2. An example of the learning outcomes for that module is shown in Figure 6.2.

BOX 6.2

CLINICAL SKILLS ASSOCIATED WITH *PHILOSOPHY AND ETHICS FOR NURSING* MODULE

- Listening/attending
- Use of silence
- Eye contact
- Proximity to patient/client

- Facial expression
- Body language and posture
- Use of touch

Core transferable skills

In line with many other universities, a number of skills considered to be core transferable skills have been identified from the literature and from policy statements developed by employing organisations and higher education institutions in the United Kingdom (Box 6.3).

BOX 6.3

CORE TRANSFERABLE SKILLS

- Self-management skills
- Teaching and learning skills
- Communication and interpersonal skills
- Problem-solving skills
- Monitoring and quality assurance skills
- Teamwork skills

Core transferable skills are identified as essential for developing effective professional practice at all levels of the programme and are included in the clinical learning outcomes for each module. At the end of the course, in addition to the successful achievement of module clinical learning outcomes, the student is required to submit a final learning statement about Core Transferable Skills achievement, together with a completed Clinical Skills Schedule record providing substantiating evidence of fitness to practise.

Although students, module lecturers and lecturers with clinical links initially reported that they needed continued support with the use of the Portfolio, after 12 months they required much less support, particularly in preparing and negotiating learning contracts. Clinical assessors are increasingly reporting greater understanding of and clarity about the curriculum, the level of competence expected of students at various stages of the course and the priorities for student learning.

Clinical Skills Schedule

The purpose of the Clinical Skills section of the Portfolio is to support and demonstrate clinical skills development throughout the course. All skills listed within the schedule are linked to the particular clinical learning outcomes of each module. The development of the Clinical Skills Schedule has been a gradual process. In light of the fears expressed regarding reduced opportunities for students to develop clinical skills (Leonard and Jowett, 1990; Robinson, 1991; Jowett *et al.*, 1992), the existing pre-registration Diploma curriculum was examined for skills content. It was recognised that the curriculum must provide a structured approach for skills learning that takes account of the reality of practice.

Students were beginning to express their concerns about their perceived lack of opportunity for skills development prior to working with patients in practice placements. The students tended to focus on tasks, procedures and skills rather than having a more holistic overview of their knowledge about nursing. This tendency for students to specify the meaning of competence only in narrowly defined terms of tasks, procedures and skills was a concern. One of the main aims of the Portfolio was to emphasise the many other elements that go to make up professional competence. At this time, there was sole reliance on students learning clinical skills within the practice area. Practical rooms had been dismantled, and skills teaching was not included in study programmes located in the educational institution. There was a lack of any structure to guide students in their learning of clinical skills in practice. A clear message coming from these students was that having to rely solely on skills learning within the practice area, with limited opportunity arising until the branch programme, caused them anxiety and distress. This was exacerbated when their apparent lack of ability to carry out tasks and procedures tended to precipitate negative comments from clinical staff, who were having to spend more time teaching them skills that they would have expected students to have acquired earlier in the programme.

Structured approach

It was recognised that students' anxiety over a lack of clinical skills might distract them and inhibit other learning in the clinical placements. Thus a more structured approach to clinical skills development was required. The first step was to identify those skills practised by professional nurses working in hospital and community settings. A survey was undertaken within the local Trusts in which students were allocated for practice placements in order to identify those clinical skills commonly practised by Registered Nurses and the frequency of practice. A self-administered questionnaire was used to gather information from a sample of clinical assessors in a variety of practice settings in the different Trusts. Based on work by Alavi *et al.* (1991), respondents were asked to indicate which skills, from a list of 67 clinical skills, they practised within the care setting and the frequency of practice. The findings were used to inform the selection and scheduling of clinical skills within a Clinical Skills Schedule that was already being developed based on the work being undertaken at St Bartholomew's School of Nursing and Midwifery (Studdy *et al.*, 1994).

A pilot study was undertaken to introduce the Clinical Skills Schedule with a cohort of students undertaking the Diploma in Higher Education Adult Nursing branch. Opportunities for learning clinical skills were scheduled within the academic study periods in addition to clinical practice placements. It was emphasised to the students that the Clinical Skills Schedule was part of a more comprehensive Portfolio of evidence of learning. Clinical skills learning is only one element of professional competence in practice. Each skill was scheduled over the 3 years, and the level of performance expected of the student by the end of the programme identified. It offered a framework for students, clinical assessors and lecturers in nursing to map progress and collect evidence of effectiveness in relation to clinical skills learning. The Clinical Skills Schedule was used to identify learning needs at the beginning of each module and prior to each placement. At the initial meeting with the clinical assessor, the student would negotiate and agree a learning contract, selecting the clinical skills to learn and the expected performance level to be achieved. For technical skills, the five levels of performance attainment described by Reilly and Oermann (1985) were used (Figure 6.3).

An initial response from some lecturers, who had not been involved with the design and development of the Clinical Skills Schedule, was that it meant more work to do with no added time in which to do it. However, the majority responded positively and felt that it offered a valuable teaching and learning framework. It would facilitate students, clinical assessors and lecturers in the structuring and sequencing of skills learning and associated theory. In addition, it would accommodate students' individual differences in learning and experience in practice, enabling students to pace their clinical skills learning according to their individual needs, circumstances and experiences while fostering a sense of responsibility in students for their own learning.

The students in the pilot study considered that the Clinical Skills Schedule provided a much-needed structure and essential guide for focusing their learning and development of clinical skills, and for learning the associated theory. The scheduling of skills teaching and associated theory was reviewed and modified throughout the study blocks and practice placements of

Level of attainment of skill	Corresponding performance criteria for technical skills only
1. • Has received instruction • Makes initial attempts at using skill	**1. IMITATION** • observed actions are followed • movements are gross • co-ordination lacks smoothness • errors are present • time and speed are based on learner needs
2. • Performs skill safely under direct supervision in a simulated care setting, for example a Skills Laboratory	**2. MANIPULATION** • written instructions are followed • co-ordination of movements is variable • accuracy is in terms of written prescription • time and speed are variable
3. • Performs skill safely under direct supervision in a care setting	**3. PRECISION** • written instructions are followed • co-ordination is at a high level • errors are minimal and do not involve critical actions • time and speed are variable
4. • Performs skill safely with minimum supervision in a care setting	**4. ARTICULATION** • a logical sequence of actions is carried out • co-ordination is at a high level • errors are generally limited • time and speed are within reasonable expectations
5. • Performs skill safely and accurately	**5. NATURALISATION** • sequence of actions is automatic • co-ordination is consistently at a high level • time and speed are within reality • performance reflects professional competence

Figure 6.3   Level of performance attainment for technical skills (adapted from Reilly and Oermann, 1985)

the whole programme. The increased contact and discussion established between students, lecturers and clinical assessors was perceived by students as increasing the support systems, providing an opportunity for the assessment of learning needs, acquiring and receiving feedback on progress, and planning experiences to facilitate clinical skills learning during both study blocks and practice placements. Students, clinical assessors and lecturers were provided with a framework for mapping progress and collecting evidence of effectiveness in relation to the acquisition of skills. It was also now possible to keep the Clinical Skills Schedule under constant review with such close collaboration with clinical assessors, and to change and to adapt the schedule in response to changes occurring within practice, adding or removing skills as necessary.

Specific skills learning is identified for each module and included in every Learning Contract. A Record of Achievement is maintained by recording the level of competence in the skills section of the Portfolio and by the presentation of valid evidence to include clinical assessor signatures on the Clinical Skills Schedule and Competence Statement sheets. This record also includes records of competence achieved during simulations in the clinical skills room scheduled within study blocks.

Through adopting an action research approach, the aim is to develop and test out in practice the clinical assessment, which includes the Portfolio. A variety of methods is being used to collect data, including regular feedback interviews with clinical assessors, lecturers and students about their experiences. In assessing progress, students, clinical assessors and module lecturers consistently report the following:

- Students and assessors need more help and more time at the beginning of the programme with writing and negotiating contracts, with evidence collection and with understanding their own and students' roles. After 12 months, the amount of help needed is much less.
- Students and clinical assessors are helped to focus learning and report that they are much clearer about what is expected of them in the learning process and the content and outcomes for learning.

- Students express confidence in having more control over negotiating and organising their learning, particularly in very busy practice placements.
- Learning Contracts provide direction to all clinical team members and help students to develop independence in learning.
- Students report increasing motivation as a result of taking more responsibility for their learning.
- Students report an increasing ability to relate the knowledge and understanding acquired during academic study to inform and enhance their learning in practice.
- Some clinical assessors are very appreciative of having access to students' reflective writing, reading and research evidence to inform their own learning.
- Some clinical assessors and students express initial anxiety about the perceived workload when introduced to the assessment instrument and tools. They regard it as a paper exercise until they have fully understood the philosophy and experienced some of the positive effects of learning in this way.

Conclusion

This chapter underlines the importance of innovative assessment strategies in facilitating both the integration of theory and practice, and the learning of clinical skills. The use of a Portfolio has proved to be an effective tool for guiding and supporting learning in practice and facilitating the formative process of developing professional competence. However, the Portfolio is only part of the process; it needs to be embedded within a structured approach to skills teaching and learning that takes account of the reality of practice.

References

Ace Project (1992) *The Assessment of Competencies in Nursing and Midwifery Education and Training.* Interim Report. Norwich: School of Education, University of East Anglia.

Alavi, C, Loh, S H and Reilly, D (1991) Reality basis for teaching psychomotor skills in a tertiary nursing curriculum. *Journal of Advanced Nursing* **16**: 957–65.

Allen, C (1992) Foundations for success. *Nursing Times* **88**(2): 20.

Argyris, C and Schön, D (1974) *Theory in Practice: Increasing Professional Effectiveness*. Mass.: Addison Wesley.

Bedford, H, Robinson, J, Schostak, L and Phillips, T (1994) *Education, Dialogue and Assessment: Creating Partnership for Improving Practice*. London: ENB.

Butterworth, T (1994) *Working in Partnership: A Collaborative Approach to Care*. Report of the Mental Health Nursing Review Team. London: HMSO.

Coates, V E and Chambers, M (1992) Evaluation of tools to assess clinical competence. *Nurse Education Today* **12**(2): 122–9.

English National Board for Nursing, Midwifery and Health Visiting (1995) *Changes to the Regulations and Guidelines for the Approval of Institutions and Courses*. Section 5: *Regulations and Guidelines Relating to Assessment*. London: ENB.

Fretwell, J (1980) An Enquiry into the Ward Learning Environment. *Nursing Times* Occasional Paper **76**(16): 69–75.

Jowett, S, Walton, I and Payne, S, (1992) *Implementing Project 2000 – An Interim Report*. Slough: NFER.

Leonard, A and Jowett, S (1990) *Project 2000: Charting the Course. A Study of the Six ENB Pilot Schemes in Pre-registration Nurse Education*. Slough: NFER.

May, N, Veitch, L, McIntosh, J and Alexander, M (1997) *Preparation for Practice: Evaluation of Nurse and Midwife Education in Scotland*. Edinburgh: National Board for Scotland.

Ogier, M (1982) *An Ideal Sister?: A Study of Leadership Style and Verbal Interactions of Ward Sisters with Nurse Learners in General Hospitals*. London: RCN.

Orton, H D (1981) *Ward Learning Climate: A Study of the Role of the Ward Sister in Relation to Student Nurse Learning on the Ward*. London: RCN.

Orton, H D (1993) *Learning Climate Project*. Sheffield: Health Research Centre, Sheffield Hallam University.

Patel, V L and Groen, G J (1991) The general and specific nature of medical expertise, a critical look. In Anders Ericson, K. and Smith, J (eds) *Towards a General Theory of Expertise, Prospects and Limits*. Cambridge: Cambridge University Press.

Phillips, T, Bedford, H, Robinson, J and Schostak, L (1994) *Education, Dialogue and Assessment: Creating Partnership for Improving Practice*. London: ENB.

Reilly, D E and Oermann, M H (1985) *The Clinical Field; Its Use in Nursing Education*. Norwalk: Appleton-Century-Croft.

Robinson, J (1991) Project 2000: the role of resistance in the process of professional growth. *Journal of Advanced Nursing* **16**: 820–4.

Royal College of Nursing (1993) *Teaching in a Different World – An RCN Discussion Document. Framework for the Future Preparation of Teachers of Nurses, Midwives and Health Visitors.* London: RCN.

Studdy, S J, Nicol, M J and Fox-Hiley, A (1994) Teaching and learning clinical skills. Part 2: Development of a teaching model and schedule of skills development. *Nurse Education Today* **14**: 186–93.

Wilson-Thomas, L (1995) Apply critical social theory to nurse education to bridge the gap between theory, research and practice. *Journal of Advanced Nursing* **21**(3): 568–75.

7

The Challenge of Primary Care

Karen Veitch

Introduction

The Northern Primary Care Development Centre was opened at the beginning of 1997. The aims of the Development Centre are reflected in the mission statement:

> To improve patient care by being an agent for change in inter-professional behaviour and working practice. The Centre will provide extensive developmental support to primary care staff and services and an inter-agency setting for primary care development and co-operative working.

Within the Centre is a Skills Laboratory, a resource that enables primary care personnel to learn clinical and communication skills to a specified level of competence before using such skills with clients. It also enables the managerial and information technology skills which support the delivery of primary care to be developed. The resource has three guiding principles. It:

- is *multidisciplinary*
- addresses *primary care* (and therefore largely those at post-basic level)
- is *regional.*

This means that the Skills Laboratory needs to be available to a wide variety of health practitioners in settings ranging from in-service training facilities to GP practices and clinics, across a large area.

Much is written about the impact of new technologies and skills in primary (or community) care, and of the benefits to clients of shorter episodes of in-patient care and the shift from secondary to primary care. However, less is written about how to make this happen and what is needed in order to support it. The word 'skill' suggests the ability to do a job well, demonstrating a level of expertise rather than merely performing an activity or task. Consequently, the key aim of the Skills Laboratory is to offer resources of the highest quality and at the leading edge in order to facilitate the acquisition of clinical and psychomotor skills and support the development of communication, IT and managerial skills. The Skills Laboratory is a concept and not just a building. This chapter describes the way in which a Skills Laboratory *with flexible walls* and a range of learning resources were developed. Future plans and developments are also discussed.

Rationale

The impetus arose from factors in three key areas:

- primary care
- advances in technology
- local context.

Primary care

There are a number of factors impacting upon primary care, which, while not necessarily exclusive to this field, often have an accumulated effect on service delivery and therefore patient/client care. There may be a significant and largely unacceptable time lag between the development of new knowledge, evidence, research or understanding and its translation into everyday practice. All healthcare professionals need to embrace the notion of life-long learning and require the means and the mechanism to support this process. The problems of practice development in primary care specialities are accentuated by staff and service diversity, isolation and geography. However, it is important that the service delivered to clients reflects the latest advances in clinical understanding, and NHS employers have a key role to play in supporting this partnership and in providing training and development opportunities (DoH, 1996).

Primary care is the bedrock of the NHS and thus offers an interesting and challenging landscape in which to plan and work. Care once confined to an acute hospital setting is now offered at or near to the client's home, being supported by advances in technology and professional practice. Yet while primary care and general practice have developed significantly over the past few years, there is a real need to develop further the infrastructure necessary to support sustained change and development, using a 'rolling programme of modernisation' (DoH, 1997).

Opportunities to develop new skills or update existing ones, particularly clinical and psychomotor skills, rely very heavily on in-service training programmes. Many are of a good standard but are weighty in terms of development, costs and staff support. Sadly, some skills are learnt on an *ad hoc* basis without means of establishing quality or appropriateness. As Mellish and Brink (1990) comment, the concept of learning by trial and error is not only wasteful of time and resources, but may also, when applied to patients, be dangerous.

Bjork (1995) argues that the shift away from hospital care requires skills in communication and collaboration as well as increased independence in nursing care within the primary care setting. However, Costain and Warner (1992) warn that there is a real danger of manpower specialities proliferating alongside every new development and that it is more constructive to retrain existing personnel. Stanley *et al.* (1993) stress that continuing medical education for GPs should recognise the educational starting point of the learners, the learning potential of professional experience and the need to develop competence continually in response to the changing demands upon primary medical care. They suggest a change in emphasis to self-directed learning based on experience, which requires a higher level of participation by individuals. A Skills Laboratory provides a resource that attempts to meet some of the difficulties experienced in practice, such as skills acquisition, the organisation of training and the provision of equipment and facilities. With the right infrastructure, the Skills Laboratory should be able to develop and expand as technology and the number of users increase.

Technology – influences on practice and learning

As highlighted earlier, the emphasis and environment for care is changing. Meads (1996) describes how community-based therapies are supported by advances in technology with the result that equipment which was once the preserve of hospital clinicians is now portable enough and cheap enough to place in GPs' surgeries. Advances in telecommunications are ushering in the telemedicine age, enabling patients in home and community settings to be 'seen' by consultants who are geographically distant from the patients.

Textual and digitised healthcare information is extensive and growing at an exponential rate. Previously unimagined opportunities now exist for the sharing of ideas, the distribution of information and collaborative problem-solving of healthcare issues and situations. It is crucial that healthcare professionals become comfortable, proficient and knowledgeable users of this form of communication (Hodson Carlton, 1995). Hodson Carlton (1996) also argues that because the new paradigm of health information delivery is one of worldwide access to resources and increased opportunities for networking and collaboration, technology must be a key component. As Hayes and Lehmann (1996) point out, the World Wide Web offers the opportunity to transmit text, pictures, sound and video to users anywhere in the world.

Local factors

A number of key people, who were familiar with many of the above issues, became aware of the potential to work collaboratively to address them. Representatives from a local Trust (Newcastle City Health), the neighbouring universities (Newcastle University and the University of Northumbria at Newcastle), local representatives of the Royal College of General Practitioners, and Newcastle and North Tyneside Health Authority formed a core group to support the development of the Northern Primary Care Development Centre.

The group wished to facilitate the development of clinical skills and provide an environment in which new skills could be learnt by utilising a Skills Laboratory approach and accessing IT, data and research. This would draw together two strands: the current drive to improve the effectiveness of healthcare, and the strengthening of primary care through the implementation of research into practice.

Development and implementation

Following the decision locally that such an initiative might be valuable, a 3-month secondment was undertaken at the end of 1996 to examine the need for and feasibility of such a development. The project was supported by Newcastle City Health NHS Trust and the University of Northumbria. It was facilitated with the help of the Skill Swap Programme, a programme that aims to match individuals with appropriate skills to identified projects, supporting them through a period of secondment. The objectives of the project were:

- the identification of a suitable physical environment for the Laboratory within the Centre
- communication and discussion with clinicians about their requirements
- the identification of similar facilities nationally and internationally
- the identification of services and facilities to be offered by the Skills Laboratory
- the identification of equipment and associated support systems
- the clarification of resource implications
- the identification of possible sources of funding

- the provision of information to the Centre's Management and Advisory Team
- the production of an implementation plan.

A questionnaire was distributed to a range of people associated with the primary healthcare field in order to determine what a Skills Laboratory might be able to achieve and how it might function. A large number of people were unfamiliar with the term 'Skills Laboratory', and many felt unable to describe what they thought it might be. However, those that did were often very accurate and demonstrated a significant insight into such a service. Much positive support was given to the need for this resource and its potential links with ongoing personal and professional development. Many felt that the ability to offer high levels of flexibility and responsiveness to problems experienced in practice was promising.

Educational resources

The Skills Laboratory services and resources need to address the needs of four key groups operating within primary care. They are:

- *nursing*: district nurses, health visitors, practice nurses, school nurses and specialist nurses
- *medicine*: GPs, GP trainees and post-graduate tutors
- *professions allied to medicine*: physiotherapists, occupational therapists, speech and language therapists, chiropodists and pharmacists
- *administration*: practice managers, receptionists and support staff.

Sessions and facilities are largely offered on a multi-disciplinary basis, and opportunities for interdisciplinary learning are strongly encouraged and supported. The range of users means that a broad range of resources is necessary. Resources can be utilised for individual use, as part of a training session within the Centre or for teaching purposes off site – flexibility is the key. As with any learning experience, facilitators within the Skills Laboratory ascertain which resources and facilities are necessary to ensure that the most appropriate strategy is used for each learning need. The level of support required may range from a simple sheet of instructions and some background information, to role play, a mannikin and a video camera. The Skills Laboratory tries to make available a wide range of resources and media to facilitate the scope of teaching and learning required.

The users are largely experienced practitioners, so reflection on clinical experience is an important aspect of the Skills Laboratory. As Spencer (1994) comments, skills learning does not take place in an intellectual vacuum, and reflection allows linkages to be made between previous experience and knowledge, meaning thus being given to what has been learnt.

Resources include:

- *Mannikins and simulators*: Lifelike simulators are available for procedures ranging from gynaecological examination to venous cannulation. They are used for teaching and assessing a wide variety of examination techniques and practical procedures.
- *Computer-assisted learning*: There are a number of very effective multimedia (CD-Rom and disk) packages available, and many more are being developed. Participants can select their own pace of instruction, repeat the material as needed and receive feedback when requested. The computers within the Skills Laboratory have been set up to run these resources with 'user guides' available as necessary. The careful consideration and assessment of these packages is important to ensure that they are appropriate and useful for the desired application. Internet access is also available within the Skills Laboratory.
- *Training packs*: These contain the elements necessary to run a training session, including, for example, a lesson plan, learning objectives, acetates, handouts and so on. They are reviewed and updated to ensure that they remain contemporary.
- *Role players/simulated patients*: Members of the local community play the roles of a patient, professional, teacher, carer, and so on to bring realism and richness to training situations by 'acting out' scenarios or situations. We have established a Role Player Agency, the APE Agency (Acting for

Professional Education), whose members are utilised exten-
sively in several practice areas. They offer practitioners the
opportunity to practise and refine their skills in a protected
but very real situation. Honest and constructive feedback is
the cornerstone of the sessions. Members of the APE Agency
will also 'perform' scripted drama, which helps to provoke
thought and discussion among participants.

• *Videos and video training packages*, of procedures, skills, system
examinations and so on have either been purchased or made
by clinicians with assistance from the Skills Laboratory.

• *Audiovisual and video production/playback facilities*, enable
participant, teacher and peer analysis and feedback. The
camera is used with the above to facilitate the teaching of
skills such as communication (consultation, breaking bad
news, history-taking and the management of aggression),
management (recruitment, appraisal and complaints) and
examination technique. The video editing suite allows
recordings of the sessions to be transferred into a 'professional' format so that they can be used and distributed as
often as necessary.

• *Clinical equipment,* such as an ECG machine and portable
suction is also available.

Personnel

The Skills Laboratory is staffed by a small core of individuals
and a flexible and diverse number of facilitators or clinical
trainers. The core staff also hold other roles and responsibilities within the Northern Primary Care Development Centre.

The Practice Development Co-ordinator is responsible for:
management of the Laboratory; development and maintenance
of the systems necessary to achieve the aims of the Laboratory; assessment and implementation of the response to training
needs; ensuring the organisation and smooth running of
teaching activities; and raising income. The Skills Laboratory
and the Northern Primary Care Development Centre both aim
to be financially self-supporting.

Two part-time technicians (audiovisual and IT) are responsible for the maintenance of such equipment as audiovisual

aids, computers and mannikins, the support of the technology used within the Laboratory, the production of in-house videos, the preparation for teaching sessions and so on.

There are two part-time receptionist/secretary posts with responsibility for receiving requests and bookings, assisting with the co-ordination of the day-to-day activities of the Laboratory and related sites, monitoring access, the maintenance of all databases within the Laboratory, assisting with the dissemination of information and so on. Together with the technicians, the receptionists work flexible hours to enable the Centre to open beyond the normal working day. This gives access to practitioners after clinic sessions as well as, importantly, to those who work part time, evenings or nights.

Clinical training and development are supported by a clinical training co-ordinator and practitioners who spend time, on a sessional basis, working within the Skills Laboratory. This ensures an accurate clinical focus and affords the opportunity to draw on the diverse range of expertise, knowledge and skills necessary to support the wide remit of the training programme. This also gives practitioners the opportunity to work in a developmental and educational role. A high level of support is given to the Skills Laboratory by the training and development staff and the Practice Team Development Unit.

Facilities

The Skills Laboratory itself is a multipurpose room, offering teaching or seminar facilities as well as computer and Internet resources. It functions as part of the wider Centre, which has a number of additional seminar rooms. The facilities are networked and have access to audiovisual technology. Educational resources are stored and displayed within the Skills Laboratory. A computerised system is used to assist with the management of resources and facilities.

The key to successful utilisation of these educational areas is flexibility in their use, that is, from small to large groups or skills demonstration to skills practice. All resources can also be transported to be used in other venues. A priority is to develop video conferencing capabilities to disseminate and utilise the Skills Laboratory resources as widely as possible.

Advantages of the Skills Laboratory

The Skills Laboratory provides a physical facility that can accommodate educational and training activities, either on site or via IT networks. A range of experts or specialists can be utilised by the Skills Laboratory to reach a large number of professionals easily. Similarly, the many and varied resources required to do this well are scarce, expensive and unlikely to be found in one discipline or institution. The Centre offers a neutral basis for a interdisciplinary education, in an environment where no professional group dominates.

The interdisciplinary basis increases the understanding and appreciation of roles. Effective healthcare is dependent on teamwork, and the key to success is mutual respect and understanding. The Centre encourages the sharing of experiences relating to operational issues within and between general practices and prevents insularity by forging links with other practices. This can also prevent 're-inventing the wheel'. Currently, one or two members of a primary healthcare team or a service are likely to go on a course; this is often expensive in terms of time, travel and fees, and often little of the information they have acquired is relayed back to colleagues in their own discipline, let alone to colleagues from other disciplines. Our intention is to increase accessibility close to the practitioner's base.

Independent access to the Centre's resources enables participants to practise, refine and maintain their competence and empowers health staff to operate in new and changing patterns of healthcare delivery. Large numbers of participants may be accommodated, and computer technology encourages participation, evokes critical thinking skills and allows control of the learning process. The Skills Laboratory can provide a valuable resource when potential course enrolment is too small to allow the cost-effective replication of facilities, departments or teaching.

A variety of agencies work within and around it to support the development of primary care in partnership with universities and primary care agencies. Significant emphasis is placed on practice development and research in primary care, addressing the need to develop a professional workforce which is able to respond to the significant shifts in care and the recognition that the professional workforce must have learning that is life-long.

Clinical skills

A list of skills relating to primary care has been drawn up, and this is supplemented by requests from practitioners and managers. The audit process is used to determine current levels and types of skill, how they are being learnt and what is still needed. This information informs the types of resource that are purchased, the facilities that are made available and the content of the programmes. As Mead (1996) comments, purchasers need training geared to future service direction, together with educational programmes that demonstrate a commitment to evidence-based healthcare, link primary and secondary healthcare and promote local priorities. Learning may focus on anatomy and physiology, disease processes and management, personal skills, examination and diagnostics, or information and communication technology.

In terms of *psychomotor skills*, the range of procedural and technical skills that are required in primary care is vast. It is difficult and time-consuming to facilitate the learning of these skills at a local level, so this aspect is consequently often neglected. Teaching is frequently implemented on a reactive or even crisis basis. The aim of the Skills Laboratory is gradually to move from a situation of reactive teaching to the proactive planned teaching of such skills. Individuals can gain 'hands-on experience', for example by using well-designed, realistic models and simulators such as soft tissue injectable trainers or pelvic examination trainers.

Communication skills, for example role play, may take place around history-taking by a nurse practitioner, the consultation skills of a GP, the negotiation skills of a Practice Manager or appraisal skills of a District Nurse.

Facilities, including computer-assisted learning, are available for the development of IT skills, decision-making and interpersonal, managerial and team-building skills as well as clinical resources relevant to practice in primary care.

Individuals using the Skills Laboratory are not undertaking a first-level professional training programme and formal assessment will therefore only be incorporated if appropriate to the learning process or for accreditation. Skills competence may be assessed, for example, by OSCE, portfolio-building, video review or self-assessment, and some computer-assisted learning packages have in-built assessment tools and learning pathways.

Evaluation of the Skills Laboratory

Evaluation of the Skills Laboratory is ongoing and operates at both a macro and a micro level in order to establish whether the services and resources of the Skills Laboratory make a difference and demonstrate continuous improvement. The resources available and the contribution of the Skills Laboratory are assessed as part of the overall evaluation of a training course or session. The Skills Laboratory has a database and resource management system that will facilitate analysis and evaluation on a broader scale. A programme of evaluation and related research will address the following issues:

- cost of its establishment and maintenance versus increased training and skills in primary care and reduced travel time and course expenditure
- practitioner and educationalist satisfaction
- an analysis of resource use and targeting as necessary
- completed research work and contributions to staff's professional portfolios
- the proportion of multiprofessional learning
- whether the technology is cost-effective
- whether the Skills Laboratory provides flexibility with support, and whether it is able to respond to the demands placed upon it.

Future developments

It is our intention to capitalise on the advantages of scale as the resources and facilities necessary to offer this type of service are significant. By co-ordinating activity on a regional or health action zone basis, a 'one-stop shop' facility can be provided to individual practitioners or teams or to satellite centres, supporting their work and ensuring the co-ordination and currency of activity and advice. The implementation of networks to support on-line access and video conferencing are planned, being phased in in line with development of the information and communication technology infrastructure within both the Skills Laboratory and the receiving sites. The additional networking of computers within the Centre and increased Internet access are also planned.

Video conferencing technology is particularly valuable in terms of primary care, lending itself readily to remote site access and to supporting speedy and interactive information transfer. It is a technology that supports the delivery of inter-active and responsive teaching and communication. Remote access will also enable skill assessment in practice environ-ments. It is anticipated that links will be formalised between other skills teaching facilities to share resources and pool exper-tise. Work on this is underway.

A help line facility is also planned, whereby support is provided to teams and individual practitioners when they have a particular type of treatment or care to deliver. This would be in the form of an agreed training pack that can be made available, video instructions, contact points with specialists or other experienced personnel, and so on. This is linked to the need to develop and maintain further information as data-bases for the Skills Laboratory that will facilitate easy access to information and networks.

Of course, the Skills Laboratory is and can only be part of the answer, and our resource is fortunate to be part of the Northern Primary Care Development Centre. Continual revi-sions will be necessary in the design, development and imple-mentation of training materials and approaches to learning as technology and practice advance and the knowledge and equip-ment status of the user changes.

References

Bjork, I T (1995) Neglected conflicts in the discipline of nursing: perceptions of the importance and value of practical skill. *Journal of Advanced Nursing* **22**: 6–12.

Carlton, K Hodson (1995) The distant learner: establishing technological healthcare resource links with the distant learner. *Computers in Nursing* **13**(5): 206–11.

Carlton, K Hodson (1996) Reengineering the learning environment linking the nursing student with the healthcare community. *Computers in Nursing* **14**(1): 19–20.

Costain, D and Warner, M (1992) *From Hospital to Home Care.* London: King's Fund Centre.

Department of Health (1996) *The National Health Service – A Service with Ambitions.* London: HMSO.

Department of Health (1997) *The New NHS Modern – Dependable.* HMSO, London.

Hayes, K A and Lehmann, C U (1996) The interactive patient: a multimedia interactive educational tool on the world wide web. *M D Computing* **13**(4): 330–4.

Meads, G (1996) *A Primary Care-led NHS – Putting It Into Practice.* Churchill Livingstone, New York.

Mellish, J M and Brink, H (1990) *Teaching the Practice of Nursing – A Text in Nursing Didactics.* Butterworth, Durban.

Spencer, J (1994) *Teaching Clinical Skills in General Practice – Report of a Pilot Project.* Newcastle: Department of Primary healthcare, University of Newcastle.

Stanley, I, Al-Shehri, A and Thomas, P (1993) Continuing education for general practice. Part 1: Experience, competence and the media of self-directed learning for established general practitioners. *British Journal of General Practice* **43**: 210–14.

8

The Way Forward

Sally Glen and Maggie Nicol

Introduction

The chapters in this book are contextualised within a period of unprecedented change in nursing. In the area of clinical skills acquisition, necessity really has been the mother of invention. Chapters 3–7 describe a number of innovative initiatives designed to address the thorny issue of clinical skills development in nursing and the difficulties associated with the provision of suitable placements for large numbers of students. The use of simulation and the concept of the practical room, which were rejected in the 1980s as being too artificial, are now re-emerging in the form of clinical skills laboratories. The following have emerged as key issues requiring debate and discussion:

- 'fitness for purpose'
- the need to balance academic and clinical needs
- the need to re-conceptualise the role of the nurse lecturer
- the need to equip nurses with the knowledge, attitude and skills necessary for life-long learning
- the demands for multiprofessional education and practice
- the influence of IT on clinical skills teaching and learning.

'Fitness for purpose'

The authors of Chapters 3, 4, 5 and 7 argue that clinical skills laboratories provide a safe learning environment in which to learn clinical skills before contact with real patients and clients, but, as the authors emphasise, they are not simply the re-invention of the practical room. The clinical skills laboratory not only provides a realistic but controlled learning environment in which clinical skills can be learnt, but also offers opportunities for experiential and self-directed learning, methods that are not usually possible in the real care setting.

It would appear that a successful clinical skills initiative requires the following:

- clear aims and objectives that are congruent with the organisation's educational philosophy
- support at the executive level, that is, by the Dean/Head of Department ensuring allocation of capital and recurrent expenditure
- an innovative and energetic individual to lead the initiative, whose job description reflects the amount of work required to set up and facilitate the development of such an initiative
- a collaborative relationship with service providers so that clinical skills laboratories are seen as a key component within a wider clinical practice framework
- sufficient lecturers who are clinically competent and clinically active
- administrative and technical staff to ensure a quality teaching and learning environment.

The authors would argue that the use of simulation is not only desirable, but has now become a necessary adjunct to clinical placements because it enables students to optimise the learning opportunities that the clinical placements offer. However, the use of simulation will never replace the need for quality, well-supervised clinical placements. Ultimately, therefore, the preparation of nurses is a shared responsibility between educators and practitioners.

A fundamental principle of nurse education is the extent to which it provides new practitioners with an appropriate foundation for practice. The phrase 'fitness for purpose' has been widely adopted in this context to describe a practitioner who has the knowledge, skills and attitudes to function as an autonomous practitioner within the present healthcare system.

However, although fitness for purpose may by the espoused objective of education programmes, the 'purpose' is becoming increasingly difficult to define.

Balancing academic and clinical needs

Nursing is not alone in grappling with the integration of the academic and practice-based aspects of the educational programme. Other vocational courses, such as teaching and social work, face similar challenges. In all these professions, the trend has been towards a more practice-based, employer-led approach, However, in a 'purchaser–provider' climate, uncertainties inevitably exist in making decisions about how we prepare nurses who are both fit for their current role and fit for the future. This leads to tension between local and national perspectives, and between short- and long-term needs; thus, as suggested in Chapter 1, there is a danger of this becoming an 'either/or' situation. There must be a recognition of the importance of equipping practitioners with a range of skills that have immediate currency at the point of registration, but equal emphasis must be given to the longer-term goals of the educational enterprise. Thus education must provide learners with a firm foundation on which, as life-long learners, they can continue to build throughout their professional careers (Rushford and Ireland, 1997). Nursing education must, of course, be employment focused, since it has to produce nurses competent to practise. However, in order to develop professionals with a repertoire of higher cognitive skills, it must remain education led rather than dominated by service requirements.

The role of the nurse lecturer

The question of whether professional nurse educators need to be a separate cadre at all (as opposed to being recruited from practitioners) can no longer be avoided. Over the past decade, there has been a good deal of interest in the development of new types of teaching appointment that, in various ways, combine the two roles of practitioner and educator. The need to review service requirements and foster collaboration between the universities and the Trusts is essential. The nurse teacher of the future should first and foremost be a practitioner, and might in future be expected to be an advanced practitioner. Certainly, the career of nurse teaching is likely to be less stable and permanent and no longer a 'job for life'. It is more likely to be characterised by a long-term employment contract consisting of a series of highly flexible, negotiable short-term role function contracts. As discussed in Chapter 2, nurse educators must remain clinical experts; otherwise, the need to have nurses teaching nursing will rightly be challenged.

Developing life-long learners

The Dearing Report (National Committee of Inquiry into Higher Education, 1997), Garrick Report (National Committee of Inquiry into Higher Education, 1997) and the government White Paper on education 'The Learning Age', (Department for Education and Employment, 1998), all emphasise the concept of life-long learning.

Healthcare organisations are seeking a multiskilled, responsive, adaptable workforce who are prepared to be life-long learners, adapting and changing as required by the organisation. Therefore, nurses need to be self-motivated and make conscious decisions about their future lives, their careers and the continuing development of their skills.

On qualifying, novice Registered Nurses require a structured and facilitated transition. Although equipped with well-developed cognitive skills, they require supervision for many clinical skills during the first year of practice. As well as these skills, there is the development of their ability to interact as part of the multidisciplinary healthcare team, representing the nursing perspective. All of this requires a nurturing and structured environment. Newly qualified nurses require clinical exposure with opportunities to debrief, to call on the clinical expertise of others and to reflect on their clinical exposure in a supportive peer environment. Nurses need to be provided with opportunities in which they not only learn how to learn from practice, but also enjoy the learning experience enough to continue learning for life. Clinical skills laboratories offer an ideal environment in which to practise skills and reflect on clinical experience away from the distractions of real clinical practice. The concept of life-long learning requires a policy framework for re-allocating nurse education resources throughout professional life. It is no longer appropriate to 'front-load' nurse education by concentrating the resources on pre-registration preparation. Educational opportunities must be provided throughout the individual's career. With the collapse of the 'conventional career', Davies (1991) suggests that nurses, in collaboration with their managers, will define their own career pathways, facilitated by the process of education and training needs analysis. A philosophy and commitment to life-long learning needs to pervade organisations (including practice areas, educational institutions and work environments), acknowledging that learning occurs in both formal and informal settings. There is a great urgency to educate nurses in the skills of case management and managed care. Nurses of the future will need to negotiate their employment and position within integrated healthcare networks (Mundt, 1997). Healthcare organisations will need to provide staff with continuing professional education to facilitate their adjustment to new roles and structures.

Nurses provide a cost-effective solution to the challenges that face our health service today: spiralling costs, the continuing advance of technology and medical science, and the inexorable shift of health services away from hospitals towards the community, in people's homes, schools, workplaces, health centres and clinics. Nurses are pragmatic and flexible, providing care across the range of clinical specialities and care environments. They have pioneered schemes such as hospital-at-home that provide flexible, relatively inexpensive nursing care in people's homes. They are leading the way in minor injuries clinics where changes in the structure of accident and emergency departments have left communities without the traditional accident and emergency services, and nurses and nurse practitioners are working directly with clients in GP surgeries, in schools and colleges, in community centres and on the streets with homeless people.

In hospitals, nurses have also changed and developed as more and more undertake roles and responsibilities previously performed only by doctors. Post-registration education therefore needs to address issues relating to the preparation of nurses in relation to their current and future development role within the care environment, thus making clinically driven education essential for practice. Advanced clinical skills are vital to the re-configuration of many nursing roles, and the provision of quality skills teaching facilities such as those described in earlier chapters provides an ideal environment for their development.

Multiprofessional practice

As illustrated in Chapters 4, 5 and 7, clinical skills acquisition offers opportunities for multiprofessional programmes of learning. These not only reduce the duplication of effort, but also introduce different world views and promote learning and the pooling of resources, thus preparing practitioners for teamwork in their professional lives. The increasing demands placed upon ever-reducing resources will force the introduction of new health service delivery models focused on the needs of the community at large. The drive for multiprofessional delivery of evidence-based care in both the primary and secondary healthcare settings will continue to challenge and blur professional boundaries.

Traditional role boundaries have in some ways been responsible for the lack of development of nursing roles in the UK. The potential for nurse clinicians as valued contributors to healthcare is restricted by the narrow interpretation by many nurses and their managers of *The Scope of Professional Practice* (UKCC, 1992), and by nurses' present lack of prescribing authority. The distinction between medicine and nursing is a political one, and the controversy surrounding the development of nurse practitioners, nurse anaesthetists and surgeons' assistants serves to illustrate this point. Very little knowledge and skill is unique to a particular profession.

As specific roles become blurred, this will lead to a point at which all the professionals involved will have to reflect on the nature of the worker who will be providing care. The kind of healthcare professional needed by the year 2010 and beyond will be different. What is needed is a fundamental challenge to all our roles, boundaries and beliefs, and, potentially, the emergence of a new professional. This is advocating a re-definition of boundaries within existing roles for all of us, including the medical profession, not the creation of a new generic 'do-all-things' worker.

Virtual skills learning

The future of nursing education is linked intricately and unquestionably to the process and outcomes of the structural reforms of the health and social care design. There will therefore be a need to substantially re-engineer curriculum design and content. In *De-schooling Society*, Illich (1973) advocated the break up of schools, colleges and universities, and the creation of new forms of learning in the home, the workplace and the community. At the time, Illich's idealistic blueprint seemed unlikely to materialise, but today it looks more possible. Illich quotes Fidel Castro, who predicted that the time would come when all Cuban universities could be closed, with the 'de-schooling' of society. This now looks a little less far-fetched than it did at the time (Blackstone, 1997).

Technology will be a key component in the educational re-design of skills teaching. Advances in computer technology have provided access to better and more affordable personal computers, and improved programming has led to new educational interactive multimedia products. The World Wide Web offers the opportunity to transmit not only text, but also pictures, sound and video in an attractively arranged format to users anywhere in the world. In future, students may be brought together to observe and practise clinical skills via personal computers linked to the Internet. This will enable them to work as a learning 'community', sharing resources, knowledge, experience and responsibility through reciprocal collaborative learning.

Technological change is likely to be even more important in bringing about the movement of education out of institutions and into the workplace and home. This shift could eventually reduce the need for institutional facilities such as classrooms and libraries (Blackstone, 1997). Clinical skills laboratories will be important for 'hands-on' practice and may need to develop as smaller satellite units linked to an instructor by technology.

The teaching and learning of clinical skills is likely to remain an important issue as professional boundaries blur and change. Clinical skills laboratories, particularly those shared between professions, appear to offer a realistic yet flexible environment for the development of professional competence. By facilitating the development and integration of psychomotor and inter-personal skills, IT skills, collaborative working skills and an orientation to life-long learning, clinical skills laboratories will play an important part in the development of the healthcare professionals of the future.

References

Blackstone, T (1997) Open all hours for the masses. *The Times Higher Education Supplement* October 17, p. 22.

Davies, C (1991) *The Collapse of the Conventional Career*. ENB Project Paper No. 1. London: ENB.

Department for Education and Employment (1998) The Learning Age: A Renaissance for a New Britain. London: HMSO.

Illich, I (1973) *Deschooling Society*. Harmondsworth: Penguin.

Mundt, M H (1997) A model for clinical learning experiences in integrated health care networks. *Journal of Nursing Education*, **36**(7): 309–16.

National Committee of Inquiry into Higher Education, Dearing (Chairman) (1997) *Higher Education in the Learning Society*. NCIHE.

National Committee of Inquiry into Higher Education, Garrick (Chairman) (1997) *Higher Education in the Learning Society: Report of the Scottish Committee*. NCIHE.

Rushford, H and Ireland, H (1997) Fit for whose purpose? The contextual forces under-pinning the provision of nurse education in the UK. *Nurse Education Today* **17**: 437–41.

United Kingdom Central Council for Nursing, Midwifery and Health Visiting (1992) *The Scope of Professional Practice*. London: UKCC.

Index